HOW HUMANITY LOST THE NATURAL WAY OF WALKING AND ENDED UP WITH POOR POSTURE AND BACK PAIN

HOW HUMANITY LOST THE NATURAL WAY OF WALKING AND ENDED UP WITH POOR POSTURE AND BACK PAIN

A COMPREHENSIVE RESEARCH INTO CONTEMPORARY AND CENTURIES OLD BOOKS AND PAINTINGS SHOWING HOW

Illustrated by
A. Markevich, M. Ribnykov, & V. Gladoun

V. GLADOUN

ARPress
ILLUMINATING IDEAS.
EMPOWERING VOICES

ARPress
45 Dan Road Suite 5
Canton MA 02021

Hotline: 1(888) 821-0229
Fax: 1(508) 545-7580

Ordering Information:

Quantity sales. Special discounts are available on quantity purchases by corporations, associations, and others. For details, contact the publisher at the address above.

Printed in the United States of America.

ISBN-13:   Softcover   979-8-89356-500-3
                eBook   979-8-89356-501-0

Library of Congress Control Number: 2024902508

CONTENTS

ANNOTATION

The author who suffered from chronic lower, mid, and upper back pain went on a dip-dive research to find out what are the roots of the problem. Surprisingly enough he discovered multiple sources such as centuries old painting and books (please see last pages of this book for the all sources) with descriptions in a great detail that back in days people naturally used to walk differently than they do it now. As a result of that natural way of walking people looked better aesthetically while walking and had multiple health benefits. You will find this information in a great detail on this book pages.

Using the healthy way of walking as a therapeutic tool along with other exercises helped the author to get to complete recovery.

ACKNOWLEDGMENTS

I wish to thank Alexander Afanasenko (Medical Doctor), Clara Malisheva (a ballet-dancer and Minsk Ballet Dance School teacher) who helped in this book's first edition preparation published in 1992, and Dr. Raymond Bartoli (Chiropractor) who helped in this book's second edition preparation. Also, special thanks go to Thomas Ellis for his invaluable and timeless medical monograph *The Human Foot..(1890)*, to George Romanes the author of The *Bodleys Afoot (1883)* to Sophia Voskresenskaya for her amazing book *The Hostess Friend (1909)*, and to many other authors and artists whose work where summoned in this book and tells us how much we lost without even noticing it when it comes to the ways of walking. Their critical findings and descriptions are referred and quoted in this book.

FOREWORD

It is my opinion (with fifteen years of experience in the field) that managing lower back pain starts at the feet and works upward. In this way, patients achieve the best results when they combine traditional medical treatment and complementary remedies. Currently, not much detailed information can be found about how to apply known complementary remedies in daily life, but this book provides a great insight. Also, the book adds one more valuable complementary remedy with the (re)discovery of a healthy way of walking.

I believe that many people would benefit from this book.

Dr. Raymond Bartoli
Chiropractor

INTRODUCTION

In my mid-twenties, I had one of the worst possible back pain problems. Actually, I had lower, mid, and upper chronic back pain. I kept visiting various doctors and health specialists, such as physicians, chiropractors, and acupuncturists on a regular basis for years. However, the medical treatment usually helped me for a day or two, and then the back pain kept reoccurring. It was a never-ending cycle.

My relatively young age led me to the conclusion that this kind of problem is not related to aging, as many people believe it is. After some time I also realized that the problem reoccurs, because the cause of it is not addressed by the medical treatments. I believed that most people have some bad habits that cause back pain to reoccur so often. Mother Nature herself could not make such a big mistake in the human body. I theorized that we must be ignoring some laws of nature. If back pain were the exception to the rule, there would be fewer people with back pain. Instead, approximately 80 percent of the world population experiences back pain at least once in their lifetimes according to Back Pain, book by R. Nordemar.

My extensive research confirmed that my hypothesis was true. In short, we walk, stand, and sit in unhealthy ways. As a result, the number of people with back pain is extremely high.

In addition, sedentary lifestyles are prevalent, meaning that many people lack adequate exercise. Without enough exercise, back muscles weaken and consequently they are unable to secure backbones properly. It allows vertebrae to misalign, leading to many different back pain problems.

To address these back problems, practitioners of conventional medicine usually recommend that patients (in addition to conventional treatments) should apply complementary methods, such as maintaining good posture in their daily activities, and performing back muscle training exercises. For instance, you can find the recommendations on the Internet at American Chiropractic Association website at http://www.acatoday.org

Good posture trains and strengthens back muscles naturally. However, even though conventional medicine widely recognizes the health benefits of good posture, most patients lack the practical experience of knowing how to implement it into their daily lives— for instance, most people do not practice good posture while walking. That is why the recommendation to use good posture does not work for most people, and they do not achieve the related health benefits, such as strengthening back muscles and potentially relieving or curing back pain. This book is focused on ways to effectively and consistently use correct posture and a healthy way of walking to produce health benefits.

Years ago, when my back pain began, I started doing back muscle training exercises and using good posture while sitting and standing. My doctor had recommended these practices to me as complementary ways of curing the back pain.

After some time these efforts helped to improve my back health dramatically. In fact, I never experienced upper or middle back pain again, however, for the next 5 years a couple of times I got lower back pain for a few days, which looks as a great improvement to me after having chronic upper, middle, and lower back pain for years and visiting doctors almost every week. This experience helped me to appreciate the complementary ways for the reason that they address the roots of the problem. However, I had a feeling that something critical among known complementary recommendations for curing back pain was still missing.

After digging into information related to the problem, I discovered that the critical point we have still missed is the natural, healthy way of walking by landing *toes first*. This, in fact, extends good standing posture to walking. In other words, this way of walking is nothing but good posture on the move. It provides excellent and natural back muscle training and provides the related health benefits. The discovered connection between ways of walking and back health is unique to the research and this book is focused mostly on it.

Back in time, at some point, the walk landing toes first was mistakenly associated with aesthetics only, and for that reason it was largely discarded and forgotten about. It was considered unnecessary. This happened around one hundred years ago or more. The worst part is that unknowingly, when that way of walking was discarded, the related health benefits were also discarded.

To make sure that the rediscovered natural way of walking would be properly implemented to result in improving health, I asked my doctor for a medical opinion. Also, I asked a ballet dancer and a ballet dance school teacher for her professional opinion regarding the walking movements. They both confirmed the findings, and helped me to prepare the first edition of this book, which was published in 1992 in Minsk, Belarus. At the same time, I did number of tests and then applied the technique to myself by using the natural, healthy way of walking more and more in my daily life as a therapeutic exercise. I had to learn how to walk again—this time properly.

This book is valuable for many people who experience back pain and those who care about posture and walking aesthetics. Years of research and tests have been summarized and placed into the pages of this book. However, be aware that applying the described techniques does not guarantee 100 percent success in curing back pain for everybody. The success depends on individual back pain cases and personal efforts. Consult your doctor (if you are not sure yet) how the technique might apply to your case of back pain (if you experience it). Nevertheless, using these natural, complementary techniques to perform regular daily activities such as walking, standing, and sitting, in addition to using standard medical treatments (such as chiropractic manipulations) is likely to help address the roots of many back problems, and therefore minimize symptoms or potentially even cure back pain. Keep in mind that in most cases, back pain problems exist only because people do not deal with them properly.

Recommended steps to address the roots of back pain are as follows:

1. Understand how back pain occurs, how weak back muscle habits work against you;

2. Learn how you can have your back muscles working for you;

3. Properly and consistently apply the techniques in your daily life.

1 What Posture and Ways of Walking Legacy Do We Have?

> *Homo erectus* (Latin: Upright man) was the first large brain hominid, which appeared around 1.8 million years ago according to anthropological science.

We can reasonably imagine that 1.8 million years ago *Homo erectus* (upright man) and even *Homo erectus* precursors before that lived in the wild, so they could not afford to have 80 percent of that population experiencing back pain. Those suffering from back pain simply would not have a chance to survive in the harsh environment. Most likely they used a posture and a walking technique that promoted back health. However, this suggestion contradicts the hunched image of a hominid (defined as *Australopithecus afarensis*) named Lucy, which has been referred to as the oldest human ancestor. The fossils were discovered in Hadar, Ethiopia in 1974, and were determined to be 3.6–3.2 million years old. Donald Johanson et al. described the hominid in the book, *Lucy: The Beginning of Humankind.* He explained that Lucy had small ape-size brain (one-third the size of contemporary humans), and claimed that she was bipedal (walked on two legs). Her leg and pelvic bones showed that she walked upright (National Geographic, #189, 1996, p. 101). In *Lucy: The Beginning of Humankind* (p. 18) Johanson stated that she was walking erect as well as contemporary people do. However, later on Johanson mentioned that Lucy's knee and pelvis suggest that she would have walked with slightly bent legs (National Geographic #189, 1996, p. 114). It appears that the Lucy's hunched image was born based on this suggestion.

On the Internet you can see the Lucy suggested images. For instance, at www.google.com click images link, type in "human evolution" (without quotation marks) as a keyword and hit the Enter button on the keyboard. It should return a number of human evolution images. In most cases Lucy is placed second from the left, next to an ape. Usually Lucy is depicted as the most hunched one. These (or similar) images were placed in almost every related school and scientific book around the world after the discovery, and now most people envision prehistoric hominids or ape-men that way. However, it later appeared that the hunched image of Lucy might be a wrong assumption for the following reasons:

1.   In *The Lucy Link* article published in *Time* magazine on Jan. 29, 1979, it was reported that Lucy was actually sick; she suffered from arthritis. This degenerative disease could cause her to walk with bent-hip, bent-knee. The image of a sick individual cannot serve as a sample of actual posture and way of walking.

2.   The *Walking tall after all* article in the *Research Intelligence* quarterly newsletter, issue 22, published by the University of Liverpool in November of 2004 describes how the university scientists used various computer simulations to answer the following questions about Lucy: How did she walk? Did she walk bent-kneed and bent-hipped like a chimp, or erect, like a human? Various computer simulations produced the following results:

-     After the Lucy walk efficiency computer simulation completed in 1998, Professor Robin Crompton concluded that in bent-knee bent-hip walking energy is stored at the knee and ankle, predicting increased heat load. With this way of walking Lucy's mechanical effectiveness would have been very low, but she could have been an effective upright walker.

-     In another simulation, Russell Savage, Li Yu, and Wang Weijie used a mechanical engineering technique to research Lucy's simulated joint motions associated with walking like a human, like a chimp, and like a human mimicking a chimp. The results indicated that Lucy could not have walked bipedal the way a chimp does, because the mechanical joint power required was nearly double that required for erect walking, and the computer model predicted a risk of overheating, so it was concluded that Lucy had almost certainly walked upright.

- Some University of Liverpool scientists decided to approach the problem from a different angle. Dr Tanya Carey collected detailed data on the physiological costs of erect and bent-hip, bent-knee walking in contemporary humans. Her study confirmed the computer model's predictions: in bent-hip, bent-knee posture the energy costs of locomotion double; the core body temperature rises so much that it is necessary to rest one and a half times as long as the time spent walking. It also indicates that with this way of walking, Lucy would have limited distances she could safely cover; that would have restricted her ability to forage for food.

3.   In 1976 at Laetoli, Tanzania, Mary Leakey discovered a trail of hominid footprints fossilized in a volcanic ash-layer (Nature Vol. 278, Mar. 22, 1978). You can see the footprints photos on the Internet, for instance, at Google images (use "Laetoli footprints" as a keyword). The footprints dated back 3.6 million years. Initially many scientists suggested that the tracks probably belong to members of the species *Australopithecus afarensis*, the hominid most famously represented by Lucy fossils, because they dated back to the same time period. Then new research called that suggestion into question. The problem is that footprints show that the feet had an arch (the bending of the sole of the foot) typical for modern humans. The researchers compared modern humans' footprints on sand with two sets of the fossil tracks and confirmed that the ancient footprints were left by individuals who had a striding bipedal walk very much like that of people today.   On

the contrary, the *A. afarensis* bone resembles that of the flat-footed apes, making it improbable that its foot had an arch like our own. Many researchers concluded that *A. afarensis* almost certainly did not walk like us or like the hominids at Laetoli:

- Latimer said that as he kneels beside the large print and lightly touches its sole, he is filled with quiet awe. It looks perfectly modern to him; 3.5 million year-old footprints are not different from ours (Gore R. *The First Steps. National Geographic*, Feb. 1997, pp. 72–99).

- However, bipedalism expert C. Owen Lovejoy of Kent State University noted that even if the *A. afarensis* foot did not have an arch, it would not mean that *A. afarensis* was incapable of humanlike walking. He continued that many modern humans are flat-footed, which makes them more prone to injury, because they lack the energy-absorptive capacities of the arch, but they walk in a perfectly normal way. In addition, Harcourt-Smith and Hilton noted that if *A. afarensis* did not make the prints, then yet undiscovered species left them, and we should consider the world's oldest who-dun-it an unsolved mystery (*Footprints to Fill, Scientific American*, August 1, 2005).

- In the article *Was Lucy a Climber*, in *Science News* #122, p. 116, Russell Tuttle, an anthropologist from the University of Chicago indicated that the Laetoli footprints that Leakey discovered in Tanzania were made by another more human species that coexisted with *A. afarensis* about 3.7 million years ago, and that it was this unknown hominid that is the direct ancestor to man. He concluded that the Hadar foot is ape-like with curved toes, whereas the footprints left in Laetoli are virtually human-like.

If this is the case, Lucy might be not related to human ancestry at all. In the search for the truth about human origin, anthropological scientists still have some contradictions and disagreements. The point is that a hunched image of a prehistoric ape-man or hominid has no scientific basis so far, because there are no proved facts. On the contrary, high arch footprints suggest upright walk and good (erect) posture, as is explained in detail in the following chapters.

2 | What Healthy Way of Walking Do We Need?

Now (after a glance at the human erect walking legacy in the previous chapter) let's see how up and how erect contemporary and "civilized" people are (quotation marks mean that walking technique has been degraded, resulting in poor back health) millions of years later.

It is remarkable that in our day there are so many faulty postures, but only one is an example of good posture, as shown in Fig. 1. Most people do not maintain good posture in their daily lives, and consequently they have squeezed chests, hanging shoulders, and protruded stomachs. How did we get to this?

A: Relaxed Poor Posture, B: Kyphosis Lordosis, C: Sway Back, D: Flat Back, E: Round Back.

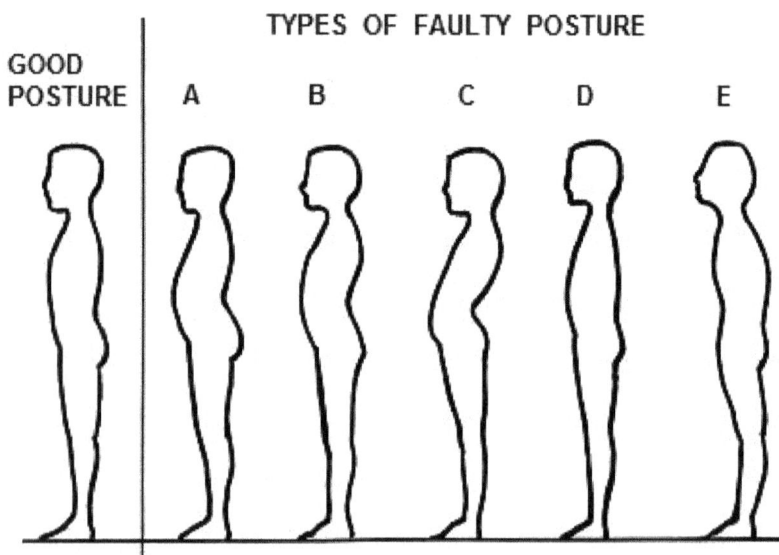

Fig. 1

I observed number of babies to determine how they learn to sit and to walk. Most of them sit straight from the very beginning, even though they do not have fully developed vertebrae curves yet. It seems that they learn to slouch later on. In the same way, most babies start to step landing toes first right from the very beginning. They learn to step in an unhealthy way landing heels first also later on—unleashing most of the primary causes of back pain and other health related problems, as it is explained in following chapters.

"Sit upright" and "stay upright"; usually these two bits of advice were all we were told about good posture during our childhoods. The same is true regarding ways of walking. Accordingly, most people think that good posture and ways of walking just have some aesthetic values, and that they are not really important for our health. As a result, most people do not pay close attention to their posture or to the directly connected subject of the way they walk. Consequently, they lose all related health benefits, and many of them experience back pain.

Multiple books and articles have been written on the subject of back pain, and the influence poor posture has on it. However, back pain still exists on such a large scale. Why? The following questions help to narrow down the problem:

1. If the primary back pain cause (weak back muscles) and the complementary remedy (using good posture for natural back muscle training) are known, why do so many people still experience back pain? The technique seems to be simple; just keeping good posture while sitting, walking, and standing will do the job. However, most people are not able to successfully apply these concepts and do not achieve the desired results.

2. Do people (even those who are not familiar with good and poor posture concepts) intentionally slouch while walking?

3. Why is back pain so prevalent in our population (as high as 80 percent of the world population)?

The answer is that a large part of the problem is that the walking technique most people use is physically incompatible with good posture; it in fact, it facilitates only poor posture. As a result, most people maintain slouch posture and consequently have weak back muscles that are unable to secure the vertebrae. This *good posture incompatibility* concept is confirmed by tests described in Chapter 5. Preliminary information and the technique details are provided in the following chapters.

Some time ago I came across a book published in 1909 named *Hostess Friend*, by Sophia Voskresenskaya. It described a walking technique landing toes first as the best way of walking for aesthetic reasons. However, in our day, most people apparently don't care much about aesthetics as it pertains to walking. People typically land heels first without thinking about how they look when they walk. Aesthetics is therefore not a reason that will likely persuade most people to walk differently.

It was a dilemma for me at first. Why does the way most people walk does not look best aesthetically? At the same time, I continued researching back pain and conducted many tests. At some point everything started to make sense; all parts of the puzzle came together. I discovered that walking landing toes first is the part we are all missing, because it promotes good posture and strengthens back muscles naturally. It added back a health benefit to the way of walking landing toes first aesthetic benefit as follows:

(1) The way of walking landing toes first looks best aesthetically.

(2) It promotes back health because it is based on good posture.

This way of walking and related health and aesthetic benefits were described in detail in the first edition of this book. Later on, while preparing the second edition of this book, I came across Thomas Ellis's medical monograph, *The Human Foot*, published in April 1890. The author completed medical research on the subject of how different ways of walking influence foot health. He proved that walking by landing toes first promotes foot health. This discovery added one more health benefit to the way of walking landing toes first (making three of them altogether):

(1) The way of walking landing toes first looks best aesthetically.

(2) It promotes back health because it is based on good posture.

(3) Also, it promotes foot health.

While the unique objective of this book is to encourage people to change the way they walk in order to promote back health, recommendations provided here also promote healthy feet as proved by Thomas Ellis, and improve walking aesthetics as described by Sophia Voskresenskaya. These benefits all come together, because what is aesthetically best is also healthiest for your back and feet. These recommendations are based on the human body's biological integrity.

It is critical to define these three benefits, because most good posture publications are focused on the posture and back pain connection only. They do not focus on thorough research of healthy walking techniques. At most they state something like this: "Walk maintaining good posture." However, this statement is inadequate, because the way of walking most people use is physically not compatible with good posture. As a result, they cannot follow through with these recommendations, and do not gain much health benefit.

Similarly, most foot health researchers are focused on ways of walking in connection with foot pain. They do not provide much information about good posture or back health. It leads to serious misconceptions because, for instance, they do not make the connection between walking techniques and back health. Similarly, why would somebody care about foot health advice if the person does not experience foot pain? For these critical reasons, this book pulls the three benefits together to consider the human body as a whole system. Following up with this point of view, the book is composed in the following order:

- Outline of back pain problems
- Basics of good posture
- Healthy walking techniques

Overview of Common Back Pain Problems

To cure back pain, we need to understand the problem first or at least get some ideas of how it works. Let's take a brief examination of common back pain problems.

What exactly is back pain? What are its symptoms?

Back pain is usually defined as deep, dull, sometimes aching or burning pain in any area of the back. However, the lower back is the most common back pain area, which is why back pain in general is often referred to as low back pain. Also, back pain could radiate from a patient's back into the buttocks and travel down the legs. Back pain can be coupled with other symptoms such as tightness in the back, neck, arms, or legs and/or numbness, which occurs when nerve impulses cannot travel properly.

Why do we experience back pain? What major problems can cause it?

1. Vertebrae misalignment

Commonly, vertebrae (spinal column) misalignment is the primary cause of back pain. Here is how it works. A properly aligned spinal column segment with attached muscles (red) is shown in Insert 1 Fig. 2. The same segment with the vertebrae misalignment depicted in Fig. 3 shows where the bottom vertebra is slightly turned to the left by a twisting move.

The misalignment strains and stretches the left side muscles shown in purple in Fig. 3. On the right side it causes muscles (shown in blue) to shrink to the shorter distance and possibly to wrench. The muscle straining, stretching, and wrenching usually causes back pain.

One more problem related to vertebrae misalignment is that if it is not fixed soon (within a day or two) the muscles can get used to the new misaligned positions. For instance, some muscles can become longer, some shorter, and sometimes slightly twisted (as shown in Fig.3). In this case, when the person later goes to a chiropractor and gets the vertebrae properly aligned as is partly shown in Fig. 2, back muscles can find themselves not used to the normally aligned position, and for that reason they can apply force toward the vertebra, and move it back to the misaligned position they had gotten used to. In this case, the problem reoccurs and back pain can become chronic.

2. Slipped disks

The slipped disk problem is somewhat similar to vertebrae misalignment, in that a spinal disk gets moved out of its normal position. One of the major problems that can cause it is that poor posture lets back muscles become weak and flabby, because those muscles do not work under normal load. Such weak muscles are unable to support the vertebrae firmly. The backbone's load redistribution occurs. That is likely to cause distress within spinal disks, leading to various other problems, including that spinal disks might be dislocated.

3. Pinching and/or Irritating Nerve Roots

Pinched and/or irritated nerve roots can cause pain and other problems in related organs, depending on which particular nerve is involved as is shown in Insert 2, Fig. 4. For example, sometimes people are not aware that the pain they feel in the stomach area, or as another example, in the heart area can be caused by a pinched nerve going from the spine to the pain area.

In addition, blood vessels also could be pinched by a misaligned vertebra or a slipped disk.

Multiple nerves go from the spinal column to different body organs as is shown in Fig. 5. This is how in the book, *De Humani Corporis Fabrica*, published in 1543, a prominent sixteenth century Belgian anatomist Andreas Vesalius depicted thirty pairs of nerves emanating from the spine. Misaligned vertebrae and slipped disks can pinch or irritate any of the nerve roots located in close proximity.

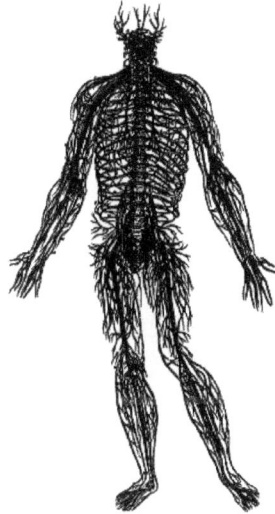

Fig. 5

4. Scoliosis

Poor posture can induce scoliosis, which is spine distortion (with back muscles in excessive tension on one side and in atrophy on the other side) and loin muscles in asymmetric tension.

5. Back muscle spasm

This problem could be attributed to a number of causes. One of the most painful is the body's natural reaction to prevent further vertebrae misalignment by straining back muscles at the moment when the body feels a dangerous move. In this case, even regular back movements could cause abrupt and sharp back pain because of strained back muscles, as the body with vertebrae misalignment attempts to prevent more misalignments. It can go in a vicious cycle: Back muscle spasms cause back pain, and automatically the body feels more misalignment danger and involves more muscle spasms as the preventing effort, which causes more pain.

6. Vertebrae disk dehydration

One of the most common causes of back pain is spinal disk dehydration. Each spinal disk contains some fluid. Insert 1, Fig. 6 shows normally hydrated spinal disk. When there is not enough fluid in the disk to keep it hydrated (as it shown in Insert 1, Fig. 7), it could cause back pain.

7. Disk degeneration

This problem's name speaks for itself, and it is attributed to poor disk condition.

In the next chapter we will explore the concept that most of these back pain problems have common roots. Understanding the underlying issues leading to back pain can provide great health benefits. These roots are related to weak back muscles, our bad habits of poor posture, and our unhealthy ways of walking.

Solutions for Common Back Pain Problems

The best approach for curing back pain is to apply standard medical procedures as quick, but short-term solutions in parallel to complementary remedies as long-term solutions. For example, whenever back pain occurs, the first thing to do is to go to a physician (emergency room in worst cases) and/or to a chiropractor as soon as possible. Physicians can help you to relive acute pain and they can provide you with muscle relaxing medicine in case of back muscle spasms.In turn, chiropractors are professional doctors of chiropractic medicine (D.C.) and they are specially trained to deal with back pain problems. For instance, they have been trained to fix vertebrae misalignments. It is critical to align the vertebrae properly as soon as possible for two reasons. The first one is to get quick relief from the back pain, and the second reason is to prevent back muscles from getting used to the misaligned position, because the back pain can became chronic that way (see the previous chapter for details). The primary purpose of the long-term solutions is to address the cause of the problem. However, *to get the long-term solutions working usually takes long time, a lot of patience, and multiple personal efforts.* The long-term solutions described in this book are based on strengthening back muscles by means of good posture, applying healthy way of walking, and back muscle training exercises.

Strengthening back muscles to secure vertebrae and slipped disks

It was shown in Insert 1 Fig. 2 and Fig. 3 how the poor condition of back muscles can cause back pain to occur and reoccur. However, the back muscle habits applied in reverse can be used for securing the vertebrae and curing back pain. Here is how it could work for you. Strong back muscles have their own habits. Should any force be applied to the vertebrae that can cause misalignment, for instance, due to abrupt twisting moves of the vertebrae, the back muscles will apply their strength to hold the spine in its used, properly aligned position.

Back muscles naturally cover vertebrae from all sides as seen in Insert 3, Fig.8 and Fig.9. When the muscles are strong, they support vertebrae from all sides, securing all back bones and spinal disks in their places. If any misaligning move occurs, they should return the affected vertebra or spinal disk back to its normal, healthy location.

Relieving pinched or irritated nerve roots

One more back pain cure is related to the cases when misaligned vertebrae or slipped disks irritate or pinch nerve roots, as is shown in Insert 2, Fig. 4. Restoring proper vertebrae alignment relieves irritated or pinched nerve roots and consequently relives the related pain or other problems.

Soothing back muscle spasms

Restoring vertebrae alignment relieves strained back muscles and consequently helps in curing the muscle spasms, which occur as abrupt muscle strains in order to prevent further vertebrae misalignments.

Curing disk dehydration, disk herniation, and disk degeneration

One more advantage strong and active back muscles can provide is related to overall muscle activity, which improves blood circulation. Let's take a look at how blood circulation in the human body is assisted by various muscle activities. First, the heart pumps out a portion of blood into arteries toward all organs and muscles. However, these efforts are enough just to bring fresh nutrients and oxygen to body cells. The cells return back into the blood their waste products and carbon dioxide. After that process blood goes into veins, for example, as it is depicted in Insert 3, Fig. 10. When the surrounding muscles flex, they squeeze the vein as is shown in Insert 3, Fig. 11. That pushes blood to both directions, but the blood vessels have inner valves that allow the flow to go one way only back to the heart.

This process supports the whole blood circulation. Accordingly, strengthening back muscles and increasing their activity improves nutrient rich, life-giving blood circulation in the back area. As a result, it better supplies each vertebra and every spine disk with all of the necessary nutrients. This helps the vertebrae to heal and to stay healthy. For instance, accordance to the American Academy of Orthopedic Surgeons website, which can be located at: http://www. aaos.org (at the time of this publication), physical activity helps to pump disk fluid back into dehydrated disks and can restore them to a normal, pain-free state.

Summarizing the solutions described above, we can see that the key to addressing common back pain problems is to develop strong and more active back muscles. It brings up the next question: *How to get strong back muscles and how to have them more active?* As mentioned above, the standard recommendations for that are the following:

1. Perform back muscle training exercises (see chapter 9);

2. Do your regular daily activities in more healthy ways, which naturally strengthens back muscles. These activities are using good posture and the healthy way of walking by landing toes first as described in the following chapters.

Note: If you experience back pain or your back pain reoccurs frequently, for instance, due to your vertebrae misalignment, which is likely for most back pain cases, you have to go to a chiropractor first to make sure that your vertebrae are properly aligned, and only after that you can exercise the muscles to strengthen them. If the misalignment reoccurs and you experience back pain, you should go to the chiropractor again to make sure that your vertebrae are realigned properly before continuing with the exercises.

This is a critical point, because as it was described above, after you get your vertebrae properly aligned, back muscles' poor habits might cause your vertebrae to return to a misaligned position very soon. To overcome this problem you might have to visit your chiropractor several times to fix the misalignment in parallel to your back muscle training until the muscles become strong enough and get used to the properly aligned position. Only then the muscles should be able to support the vertebrae securely.

Performing back muscle exercises

For number of back muscle training exercises, please see chapter 9. Your chiropractor can provide you with more of them if you need. Also, you can find many exercises at the American chiropractor association web site located at: http://www.acatoday.org

Using good posture and the healthy way of walking in daily life

As discussed previously, using good posture and the healthy way of walking in daily life can actively strengthen back muscles. The main idea (described in many books and multiple web sites) is that we need to use good posture for sitting, standing, and walking. For instance, if a person mostly lies back in a chair or seat with slouch posture, his or her back muscles are typically relaxed. Another unhealthy habit example is when while sitting, somebody supports his or her torso by placing elbows on a desk. Then, the back muscles are not active enough because the arms do the supporting job. These are just two of many lazy tricks people use and consequently keep their back muscles relaxed and not active most of the time. On the other hand, good posture ensures that back muscles work actively. Accordingly, the goal is to apply good posture for sitting, standing, and walking to have back muscles work actively, which strengthens them naturally and provides many other health benefits.

The health benefits and techniques for achieving good posture and the healthy way of walking are described in detail in the following chapters.

Poor posture is unattractive for personal appearance. For example, many people perceive individuals with good posture as interesting and alert, as is shown in Fig. 12, while people with slouch posture are viewed as awkward, as is shown in Fig. 13. In other words, poor posture is socially undesirable. Good posture (shown in Fig. 12) is the natural position the body assumes when all body parts are in total balance. This is the reason why good posture is also called *neutral*. Another reason is that around 90 percent of body muscles relax and most importantly, among the 10 percent of the muscles working are back muscles—exactly the muscles that must be active for a healthy back. Correct posture involves proper pelvis, abdomen, rib cage, shoulders, neck, and head alignment. To a large extent, good posture is a matter of holding in one's abdomen, and also holding shoulders back and down in order to stand straight up without slouch appearance.

Good posture is shown in Fig. 12. Poor posture is depicted in Fig. 13, and it can be described as slouch body position with stuck-out abdomen and squeezed chest.

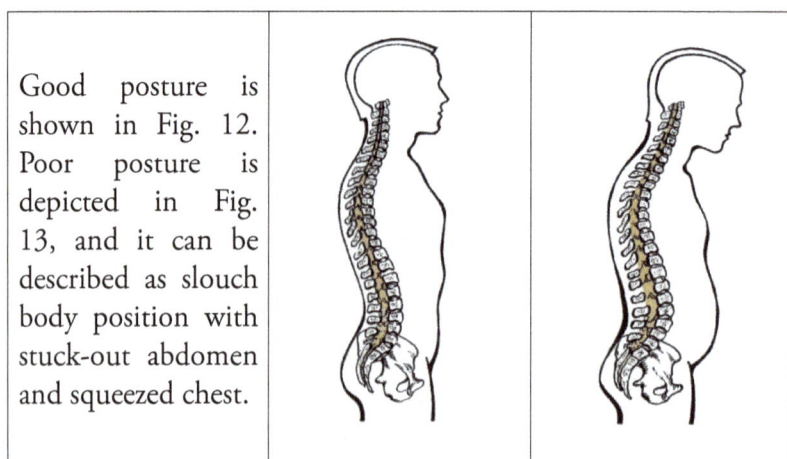

Fig. 12   Fig. 13

When poor posture is assumed, back muscles do not maintain the torso in balance and mostly relaxed. Accordingly, poor posture unevenly distributes the weight of body parts, and as a result it puts much stress on some joints, which can stretch or tear ligaments and tendons. Poor posture also puts uneven pressure on each vertebra and the disks between them, which can cause vertebrae misalignment, slipped disks, and other back pain problems. It makes maintaining good posture a vital goal.

Good posture is the maintenance of the normal spine curvature without leaning forward or backward. In other words, the spine should not be over-curved or under-curved. Otherwise, body parts will not be in balance. The balance allows back muscles to work properly without over-strain or under-strain. Let's look in detail at the following question: What happens if good posture is not maintained in one's daily life, and accordingly his or her back muscles are not usually active? To answer this question let's recall the following facts. What happens when people do not walk for a long time? For instance, some astronauts did not walk for more than two months because of long flights. What happened to their leg muscles and their ability to walk? Their leg muscles became weak, and they were unable to walk normally for weeks after landing, even though they had done many exercises for the duration of the flights. The same is true for back muscles. If we do not use them actively, for instance, to maintain good posture, they become weak.

In this connection, most people use their elbows placed on desks to support their upper body weight. Also, they usually lie back in chairs. Most people do not sit straight with good posture. Another lazy trick people use for standing to avoid efforts to keep good posture is to lean on something using different body parts, for instance, the pelvis or shoulders. The problem is that by doing that they do not use their back muscles actively, and they miss the natural opportunity to exercise them. As a result most people's back muscles are poorly conditioned, and for that reason, the muscles are unable to secure their spinal columns. No wonder that up to

80 percent of the world population experience back pain at some point in their lives.

How to Assume Good Posture and Develop the Healthy Habits of Good Posture

Good posture (sometimes defined as neutral, or nominal, or proper) can be assumed by one of the following ways:

Way 1:

Back health specialists' common practice in teaching good posture is to instruct patients to stand with their backs against a wall, pressing their pelvis, heels, spine, shoulders, and back of the head against the wall (with arms hang freely). A flat door also can be used for this purpose. You need to stand tall with your chin slightly tucked in. Rise up your chest, inhale more air, pull in your abdomen, and tighten your buttock muscles. This position is said to simulate good posture, as is shown on Fig. 14.

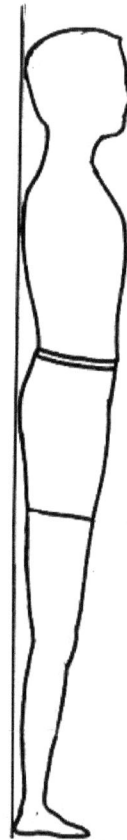

Fig. 14

Way 2:

Make sure that your ear, the shoulder joint, and the hip joint are stacked in a straight line as shown in Fig. 15.

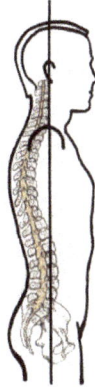

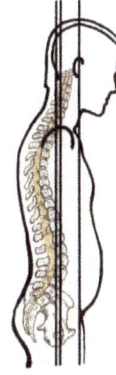

Fig. 15   Fig. 16

To assume good posture using this method, you might need somebody's assistance. To simulate the line, another person can use a plumb line, which is essentially a string with a weight at the end. When posture is poor, the ear, the shoulder joint, and the hip joint are not aligned. Three vertical lines drown through them would not come together, as is shown on Fig. 16.

Way 3:

This way of assuming good posture is essentially the same as Way 1 or Way 2, but without the wall or somebody's assistance. When you become more familiar with the technique, you should be able to assume good posture by this way 3. This skill is essential for learning healthy way of walking techniques. Here is how to use the technique and how to check for good posture:

1. Assume good posture following the technique from the Way 3. Your body weight should be kept in the middle of your feet.

2. Perform this good posture checking test: Lean a little bit forward without losing good posture, and at the same time slowly move

your body weight from the middle of the feet to your toes, raise your chest up a little bit, and inhale more air.

3. When the weight moved to your toes, you should be able to rise on your toes without losing your good posture or balance (no falling forward or backward).

More good posture health benefits

Let's take one more look at good posture depicted in Fig. 12. The chest is raised up, which lets more air get into the lungs while breathing. Otherwise, when poor posture is assumed, as is shown in Fig. 13, the chest is squeezed, and for that reason the lungs have to work in a tight breathing space. As a result, the person's blood does not receive as much oxygen as it should. Also, the person's heart must work in the squeezed room too. You do not need to be a doctor to understand that this is not healthy.

Who benefits from poor posture? This is only the stomach, because the stomach can freely expand. It also pulls forward the lower vertebrae (called lumbar) shown on Insert 4 Fig. 17 out of normal position (shown on Insert 4 Fig. 18) giving it more sharp curve, as is shown on Insert 4 Fig. 19. This makes the lumbar more vulnerable to misalignments and spine disk slipping. As a consequence, most back pain problems occur in the lower back area.

On the other hand, good posture provides the whole arrangement vice versa. It tightens in the belly, smoothes the lumbar curve, raises up the chest, giving more room for the heart and lungs to work— which is one more excellent reason to maintain good posture in addition to addressing the roots of back pain problems.

To summarize, good posture is an effective way to address most back pain problems and get related health benefits. However, the problem is that the good posture is physically not compatible with the ways most people walk. More about this will be discussed in the following chapter.

Your standing technique controls your posture, making it either good or poor.

The following tests demonstrate that we physically cannot stand assuming good posture, if we keep our body weight on our heels.

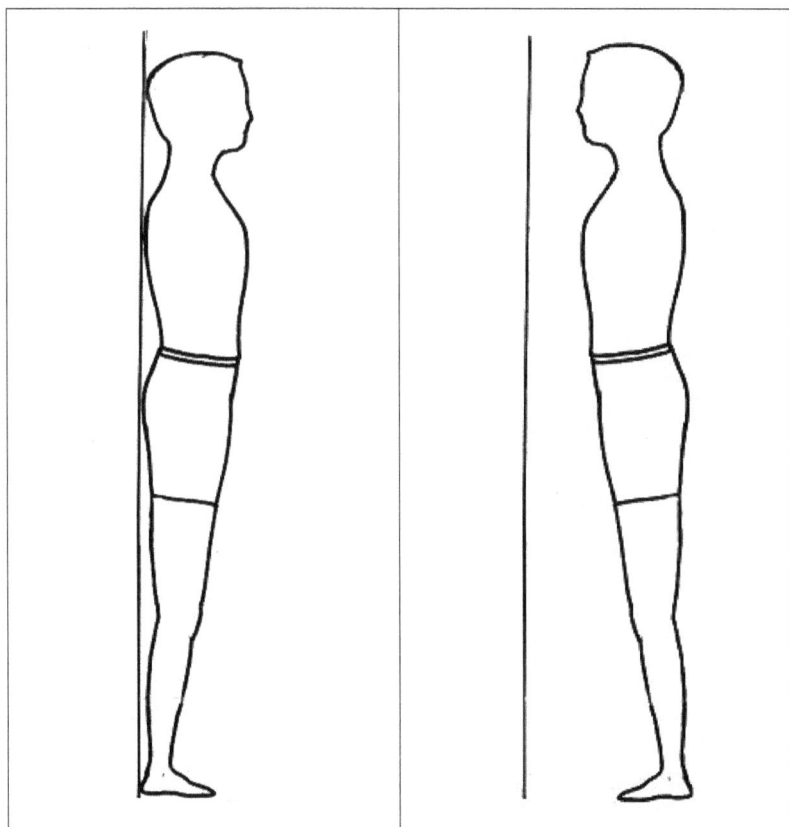

Fig. 20   Fig. 21

Test 1

1. Stand at a wall (or a flat door) and assume good posture as shown in Fig. 20 (pressing the pelvis, heels, spine, shoulders, and back of the head against the wall).

2. Rise on your toes. Note that you are still able to maintain good posture.

3. Return to the Step 1 position and try to raise your toes up. Note: To be able to rise your toes up, you have to move your body weight to your heels. It breaks good posture; your body looses balance and tends to fall forward.

Test 2

1. Assume good posture as is shown in Fig 20 above.

2. Step approximately 10 to 15 inches forward using many tiny steps (a few inches each to ensure keeping good posture) and slowly turn around to face the wall as shown in Fig. 21. Continue to maintain good posture. Note the distance between your nose and the wall. You should keep the distance the same for the whole test. Please be careful in doing the following steps. Perform them very slowly to make sure you do not hit the wall with your nose or with other parts of the body.

3. Move the center of your body weight to your toes. Slowly raise your chest further up and inhale more air. Then raise your body onto your toes. Note that you are still able to keep good posture. The distance to the wall should still be the same.

4. Slowly descend back to your feet. Keep the distance between your nose and the wall the same, and slowly move the center of your body weight backward from your toes to your heels. Note that you have to move the middle part of your body backward to be able to keep the same distance from your nose to the wall. Now slowly try to raise your toes up from the floor (even a little

bit) to ensure that your body weight is on your heels. Note, that keeping good posture is impossible now.

This is the root of the problem with the unhealthy way of walking, landing heels first. *We are physically unable to maintain good posture when our body weight is on our heels.* Walking and landing heels first guarantees keeping your body weight on your heels, and as a result it ensures assuming poor posture. This promotes various back pain disorders. However, most people habitually walk by landing heels first.. A solution to the problem is in incorporating good posture and the technique of walking by landing toes first into one healthy way of walking.

Summary:

Good posture helps to strengthen back muscles naturally, which is critical for overcoming most common back pain problems. Accordingly, the healthy way of walking strengthens back muscles, because it uses good posture actively. In other words, this way of walking strengthens back muscles better than by just using good posture for sitting and standing. For instance, in addition to keeping good posture at every step in walking, the activity of the back muscles provides twisting movements of the vertebrae. It trains and strengthens the back muscles naturally. (The back muscle samples are shown on Insert 1, Figs. 2– 3, and Insert 3, Fig. 8, and Fig. 9).

What is known about walking? Let's look into some books.

Walking is an activity everybody seems to know about. At a glance, its technique looks simple and familiar. However, if you try to find detailed information about which way of walking is more natural or healthy, you will find a lot of confusion on that topic. For example, some books claim that the right way of walking is to step landing heels first, but a number of others claim the opposite—that toes should land first. For instance, the following books (some about people and some about mammals in general, but they describe walking technique for people too) address the walk landing heels first:

1. *Teaching for Outcomes in Elementary Physical Education* by Christine J. Hopple, 1995, p. 86;

2. *Your Active Child* by Rae Pica, 2003, p. 118;

3. *A Field Guide to Mammal Tracking in North America* by James C. Halfpenny, Elizabeth Biesiot, 1986, p. 10;

4. *Skulls and Bones: A Guide to the Skeletal Structures and Behavior of North American Mammals* by Glen Searfoss, 1995, p. 114.

The following books focus on the way of walking landing toes first:

1. *Walk Shaping: Indoors Or Out, 6 Weeks to a Better Body* by Gary Yanker, 1995, p. 72;

2. *Creative Leadership in Recreation* by Howard Gorby Danford, 1964, p. 257;

3. *Skill Development Through Games and Rhythmic Activities* by Charles Nagel, Fredricka Moore, 1966, p. 118;

4. *Walking: A Complete Guide to the Complete Exercise* by Casey Meyers, 1992, p. 98;

5. *The Human Foot: Its Form and Structure, Functions and Clothing* by Thomas Ellis, 1890, p. 51;

6. *The Hostess Friend* by Sophia Voskresenskaya, 1909.

To complicate matters further, the following books describe both ways mentioned above:

1. *Handbook of Brain and Behavior in Human Development* by Alex Feddle Kalverboer et all., 1993, p. 506;

2. *British Manly Exercises: Containing Rowing and Sailing, Riding & Driving* by Donald Walker, 1836, pp. 24–26;

3. *The Bodley Books* by Scudder Horace Elisha, 1879, pp. 89– 91.

Also, if you search the Internet using the following search keys "walk landing heels first," "walk landing toes first" and such, you will see a lot of contradictions too. So many different opinions exist on what seems to be a simple subject that is known to everybody—walking. However, when it comes to running techniques, the authors of the books mentioned above all agree that the right way of running is to land toes first.

To whom shall we listen? Who among the authors of these books should we expect to be most knowledgeable and experienced in walking?

To define the best way of walking, let's look into the problem from this point of view: "What is healthier and more natural?" In this connection, the first question is: "To whom shall we listen?" Let's use the scientific approach, which is to base a theory on facts. Many contemporary authors of the books mentioned above do not give us any facts or reasons why they think that the walking technique they describe is best. Statements about ways of walking without good reasons and facts sound to me like this: "This way is right and it is the best because I do it that way." This is an opinion, but not a fact. Accordingly, such statements don't have a virtue to be called a truth from scientific point of view. In other words, facts and tests must prove the opinions right or wrong and the techniques healthy or unhealthy. On the other hand, a number of books published around one hundred or more years ago provided good scientific (including medical) reasons and facts about walking techniques. Why? Around, the 1900s or earlier, people had to walk much more than we do now, because transportation options were not developed to the extent they are today. For instance, Thomas Ellis, in his medical monograph "The Human Foot," which was published in the April 1890 issue of *Wood's Medical and Surgical Monographs* (Vol.6, Number 1, p. 50) mentioned that at that time solders walked daily up to 20,000 steps per foot, making it up to 40,000 steps per day altogether. This is very impressive walking experience. Good walking technique was essential for them, because doing it wrong caused severe foot sores, foot injuries, and pain. Back then it was the primary reason for doing extensive medical research on the subject to define the healthy and unhealthy ways of walking. As a result, books published on the subject around that time deserve very close attention.

Taking all of that into consideration, let's look into some facts about different walking techniques. The facts described below prove that landing heels first while walking is unhealthy and unnatural, and that landing toes first while walking is healthy and natural.

More Anthropological References: What did two prominent scientific/medical researchers discover at the end of nineteenth and beginning of the twentieth century? What ability did Mother Nature build into the human foot?

George John Romanes, in his book *Darwin and After Darwin,* published 1910, on p. 182 brought up an interesting point about mammalian feet digitigrade modification as compared to reptiles and early mammals. To understand this point better, we should know a few related scientific definitions. Thomas Ellis provided them in the book, *The Human Foot* mentioned before. On p. 19 he explained that: "Mammalian animals are classified, as regards to their mode of progression, according to varied forms of the foot.

Pinnigrade, if it be expanded like a fin, or *pinna*, as in the seal, where it is adapted for moving in water. *Plantigrade*, where the whole foot lies flat on the ground, forming a sole or *planta*, as in the bear; *Digitigrade*, where the tarsal bones are raised so that the weight comes upon the digits or some of them, as in the dog; *Unguiculate*, where the whole weight comes onto one digit, and the nail or unguis is expanded into a hoof, as in the horse. Man is classed as plantigrade, but in every step as he walks he becomes, alternately, digitigrade; in running he remains so. This feature in man is unique."

The point George Romanes brought up is: "The digitigrade modification necessitated a change of structural plan to the extent of raising the wrist and ankle joints off the ground, so as to make the quadruped walk on its fingers and toes. We meet with an interesting case of this transition in the existing hare, which while at rest supports itself on the whole hind foot after the manner of a plantigrade animal, but when running does so upon the ends of its toes, after the manner of a digitigrade animal." This point leads us to a better understanding of the *human foot, which also has this structure built-in.* Humans can switch between digitigrade and plantigrade movements.

Going back to *The Human Foot*, on p. 29 the author explains that, "One of the most interesting and important movements which the muscles' action on the foot are designed to effect is to raise it to the tip-toe position, or, in other words, to change it from the plantigrade to digitigrade form. *The whole of the weight then falls on the anterior pillar of the arch alone. How this is done, not only without damage but rather with increased strength to that structure, must be fully comprehended if the mechanism of the foot is to be understood.* The action is sometimes described as that of a lever of the first order, where the power of the muscles of the calf acts on the heel, and, through the fulcrum formed by the leg, on the weight supplied by the resistance of the ground against the toes. Another and a better way of putting it is that the lever is of the second order, the weight being that of the body, while the fulcrum is supplied by the toes."

Inserts 5–8 show how T. Ellis depicted various parts of this structure in detail to explain how it works. In addition he provided two figures (shown below) for the general view.

"Fig. 27 shows the tendons of one muscle only crossing the sole from end to end, all else being, for the sake of clearness, removed. This, the tendon of the flexor longus pollicis, has, to the arch of the foot which it subtends, the relation of a chord to an arc, of a bow-string to a bow. Now this arch, or arc, or bow, is made of flexible material." (T. Ellis Fig. 27)

"Fig. 28 shows the effect of muscular action in throwing up the arch and is to Fig. 27…

1 is the flexor longus pollicia,

2 the tibialie pasticus, and

3 the combined calf muscles."

(T. Ellis Fig. 28)

Thomas Ellis explained:

In either view there is an essential difference from ordinary levers: the power of attached to the leg, i.e., to the fulcrum or to the weight, according as the action is regarded as that of a lever of the first or of the second order. Both views are, however, liable to mislead. It is usual to give the combined muscle acting on the heel as the power by which the body is raised to tip-toe as if it were the only power. One who writes with the highest authority says, in a book intended for general readers, 'The muscle which acts upon the heel is one of the largest and most powerful in the body, and well it may be, for in raising the heel it has to raise the whole weight of the body.' This is misleading and inaccurate. If the foot be taken when at rest, no tendons can be felt behind the ankles; when the body rises to tip-toe they start out on either side. The most prominent on the inner side is the flexor longus pollicis (Latin), on the outer the peroneus longus. Those tendons which are deeper are also tightened; the flexor longus digitorum and the tibiales pasticus on the one side, and the peroneus brevis on the other. Now all these muscles are strong, their combined strength is enormous and although they do not act at the same advantage as the calf muscle, which acts on the projecting or lever-like heel, they do exercise a very great influence in bringing the leg and foot toward a continuous straight line, which is the essence of the tip-toe movement. Take the first-named only; the flexor longus pollicis is so strong that it may be trained to bear the weight of the body itself, as in the stage dancer, who will support himself, or more generally herself, literally on the great toe. Though incapable in most persons of anything like such a feat as this, the muscle in question is, in all good feet, very strong.

To prove this point, Thomas Ellis provided the following story that he encountered in his medical practice:

Of my long-entertained view that the influence of the calf muscle in walking has been over-rated, and that of the other muscles under-rated, I have recently had a striking illustration. A young gentleman, able to take his share in rough games at a public school, and to do a long day's shooting with his farther, an excellent walker, has, on one side, no calf muscle at all. It had been paralyzed in infancy, and neither it nor the tendo achillis has developed; the latter is, in fact, a mere attenuated ligament, contrasting strongly with the specially developed tendon on the other side. Here an extra development of the remaining muscles of the same side and of those of the opposite foot and leg have almost completely compensated for the deficiency, so that the subject and his friends are hardly conscious of any defect. Had the deficiency existed in both legs it would have been serious indeed.

The mechanism of rising to tip-toe consists in an elevation of the heel by the great calf muscle acting upon it, assisted by the concurrent action of the groups of muscles whose tendons pass down behind either ankle. These latter, which move the foot or the toes, when those parts are free to move, move the body on the foot when the foot is fixed. To say that the body is raised by the calf muscle action on the heel (a statement often made), is an incomplete and misleading description. The same action continued and effected with sufficient vigor propels the body forward, whether for purpose of walking, running, hopping, or jumping.

But so that the heel be raised does it very much matter how it is done? The answer to this will appear from the following considerations: If, then, the arch be yielding, and the muscle acting on this tendon be strong, both of which facts are indisputable, the action of the muscle must brace up the arch as certainly as tightening a bow-string increases the convexity of the bow in diminishing the distance between the ends of it. (*The Human Foot*, p. 50. Also, see Insert 7, Plate 3, Fig. 8 for details.)

The drawings show how the human foot has a built-in mechanism for rising to the toes, "when the whole weight falls on the anterior pillar of the arch, it is done not only without damage, but rather with increased strength," according to Tomas Ellis *The Human Foot, p. 29.* Please see strong foot bones, foot arch mechanism, strong foot ligaments, and three levels of muscles in the human foot shown in Inserts 5–8.

All of the observations conducted by such prominent researchers as Thomas Ellis and George Romanes proved that the *ability to rise on toes is not an accidental, but a comprehensive and powerful functionality naturally built into the human foot.*

Another excellent point Thomas Ellis brought up is that *ways of walking influence foot health.* First of all, here is how a good way of walking is described in *The Human Foot* on p. 39: "In walking toes should be pointed downward so they and not the heel should first touch the ground." And further more: "*It is the natural walk* at least for the highest types of savages." (*The Human Foot*, p. 51). "For instance, natives in America walked landing their toes first." Also, on pp. 51–52 a more detailed explanation is provided:

In good walking, the toes should reach the ground first: they are the organs of feeling: it is for them to literally feel the ground. In discussing the question, which part of the foot should reach it first, it must be remembered that use of the shoes cannot be pre-supposed. Man must be considered as going barefooted if we are to discover the best mode of walking. In the savage state, the foot never has hardness at all comparable to the hoofs of animals; it is not to the savage a matter of indifference what he treads on. Now let it be supposed that he is walking where he is liable to encounter sharp objects hidden, it may be by verdure. If such an object be felt by the toes in pointing the foot forward, it is possible to avoid it by withdrawing or diverting the toes while still holding the ground with the other foot. If there be no impediment, if good foot-hold for the toes and front part of the foot be found, it will afford a bearing. On this bearing the walker can spring if any sharp object comes in contact with the sole of the hinder part of the foot. Moreover, the heel, coming last, is the least sensitive part of the sole. On the other hand, if the heel reaches the ground first, it is a poor guide as to the nature of the foothold. Let us assume it to have come on a good surface, but that the point where the tread will fall is occupied by a sharp object unsuspected. In that case, when the weight of the body falls on it, recovery is impossible: one can't spring backward on to the heel as one can forward on to the toes.

Thomas Ellis explained that in most cases a *flat-foot is a consequence of the bad way of walking landing heels first.* On the other hand, *the good way of walking landing toes first helps feet to shape properly.* He provided the following examples: "Among races going barefoot the practice seems to vary. The Arabs, who have finely developed feet, point the toes downward, while some of the flat-footed inhabitants of India are said to bring the heel first to the ground." (*The Human Foot*, p. 53)

T. Ellis described medical cases where a damaged or injured foot was restored by using the walk landing toes first and rising to tip-toes exercises. Very remarkable is his own case. A horse stepped on his foot and severely flattened it. It took him many months and much effort, such as rising to tip-toe exercises and using the way of walking landing toes first to have the damaged foot shape restored from flat to arch. Eventually, this remarkable fact encouraged him to study the human foot so deeply. (For details about this case please see *The Human Foot*, pp. 64 –70).

More facts and reasons to use the walking technique landing toes firsts. Good and bad things shoes brought to us.

If you try to walk barefoot on the ground, you might notice that the walk landing heels first hurts more than landing toes first. It happens because the former way is essentially pounding the ground with your heels. Also, this way is more painful when you step on small rocks and other rough objects. The other way (landing toes first) has toes working as shock absorbers, as many muscles are involved in the landing. Nature built toes to work that way as described previously.

This natural technique worked fine for most people until durable shoes were invented. After that, it appeared that there was no need to step as carefully as barefoot people or people with light shoes had stepped before. Some people tried to stick with the old tradition for some time for aesthetic reasons. Nevertheless, most people have walked carelessly since then. However, this careless walking comes with a price, which is poor posture and consequently back pain.

In the process of exploring ways to walk the following question might arise: "What is the purpose of the heel?" Thomas Ellis explained:

It is fitted with a firm and at the same time soft pad covered with a thick skin, and is so adapted better than any other part of the foot for contact with the ground. Is this a reason for believing that the weight of the body is intended to fall upon it in walking? We are told that to place the foot almost flat on the ground is mistake, as the body losses in part the advantage of the 'buffer-like mechanism' of the toe. This would be pertinent if the construction of the heel were not otherwise explained. As it is, there is nothing in it to outweigh reasons for believing that the heel is intended for a different purpose. The heel is admirably adapted for sustaining the weight of the body, which, in the position of standing at ease, falls mainly upon it, and is by it transmitted to the ground. For this purpose a soft covering is very desirable, which consideration alone is sufficient to account for the cushion-like pad beneath the heel, hardly, however, to be compared to a buffer. (The Human Foot, p. 53. Also, please see Insert 7, Plate 3, Fig. 9 and Insert 7, Plate 5, Fig. 16 for details).

Walking landing heels first guaranties having poor posture.

Tests described in the beginning of this chapter have shown that we are physically unable to assume good posture if we keep the body weight on our heels. Accordingly, walking by landing heels first ensures keeping the body weight on heels, and as a result, guaranties having poor posture. This happens because all body parts and the body mechanical movements are interconnected. Changes in one part automatically cause changes in other parts. On the other hand, the walking technique landing toes first ensures keeping the body weight on our toes, which invokes assuming good posture.

Walking landing heels first causes pain in heel and leg bones.

Walking landing heels first (especially walking that way for a long time) causes pain in heel and leg bones, because every step gives them a pounding shock. The pounding propagates from heels directly to leg bones. On the other hand, walking landing toes first technique works quite the opposite. Numerous muscles help to absorb the shock. It works as a buffer, making the foot landing smooth.

Poor walking technique irritates heel nerves.

The heel pounding (because of landing heels first) irritates heel nerves, which can cause heel and leg pain.

Walking by landing heels first shapes leg muscles poorly.

The walking technique of landing heels first does not completely employ the calf and other foot muscles related to the rising on toes mechanism. As a consequence, many people do not have these muscles properly trained and shaped. On the other hand, the walking technique of landing toes first better strengthens and shapes these muscles. More details on this can be found in Chapter 8: Walking and Posture Aesthetics.

Better calf and other muscle activity improves blood circulation in legs.

One more good reason for the calf and other muscles to engage in foot rising activity is the resulting improved blood circulation. On Insert 3, Fig. 10 and Fig. 11 it is shown how the muscle activity helps to pump blood in the body. In this connection, better leg muscle activity pushes more blood on the way back to the heart, improving the whole blood circulation.

Walking landing heels first causes heel skin to become more dry and rough.

Another problem with walking by landing heels first is that heel skin becomes more dry and coarse, because heels experience harsh friction when a foot lands on it first. On the other hand, when a foot lands on the toes first there is no such rough friction present because of the foot-toe buffer-like mechanism.

Squeezed chest (which is a consequence of poor posture and unhealthy way of walking) leaves less space for the heart and lungs to work, but the stomach has plenty room to expand.

In Fig. 13 it was shown how the chest is squeezed when a person has poor posture. Let's compare it to the chest depicted on Fig. 12 when the person assumes good posture. This is one of the most critical points. I saw on the Internet that some people are shocked by the fact that our feet have been distorted by shoes (as compared to what they would be naturally without using any shoes). I have a message for them: *Our distorted feet are a small problem compared to what poor posture and unhealthy ways of walking distort in our bodies.* For example, in the squeezed chest our lungs cannot breathe in their full capacity. Accordingly, less oxygen gets into blood, causing some body hypoxia (oxygen deficiency reaching the tissues of the body). The hypoxia could cause any of the body parts to suffer. For instance, brain hypoxia imprints on central nervous system functionality. It can cause fatigability, excitability, headache, insomnia, and so on. Also, the compressed chest leaves less space for heart to work, so the heart works within a squeezed environment too. This all occurs in addition to back pain problems.

Healthy way of walking improves emotional state.

An interesting point is that muscle activity and our emotional state are interconnected. A. Alekseev M. D. pointed out that the connection between brain and skeletal muscles works bi-directionally. It is not only that the nervous system affects muscle tone, but muscles, in turn, influence the nervous system. For instance, deliberately strained skeletal muscles tense one's nervous system, and to the contrary, deliberately relaxed skeletal muscles relax the nervous system (Alekseev, A., *Science and Life*, 1979, #4). In this connection, mincing, loose, and waddle ways of walking influence one's nervous system state accordingly. On the other hand, a good, diligent way of walking tunes the nervous system better.

The way of walking landing heels first is less stable.

One more valid point is that landing the heels first way of walking is less stable compare to landing the toes first. This is because in the former, one's body weight is shifted to the heels. I noticed that many people have learned it the hard way while walking on slippery surfaces such as icy pavements or wet floors. Also, I observed on many occasions that the same people intuitively began to step landing their toes first for some time right after the fall. The walking by landing toes first technique naturally moves the body weight forward to the point of the foot-hold, making the whole body more balanced and the walk more stable.

Note: Most people walk landing toes first when going up or down stairs.

Summary:

- Ability to rise on toes is not accidental, but a natural complex system, which is built-into the human foot;
- The way of walking by landing heels first ensures assuming poor posture;
- Durable shoes let people use a simplified, but unhealthy walking technique of landing the heels first;
- Walking techniques controls body posture to make it good or poor;
- Pounding heels in the way of walking by landing heels first causes pain in heels and leg bones;

- The poor way of walking irritates heel nerves;
- Landing heels first walk poorly shapes leg muscles;
- Better calf and other related muscle activity is found in the healthy way of walking by landing toes first;
- Walking by landing toes first improves blood circulation in legs;
- The poor way of walking causes heel skin to become more dry and rough;
- Landing heels first ensures poor posture, which squeezes the chest and leaves less space for the heart to work and lungs to breath, but the stomach has plenty room to expand;
- The healthy way of walking improves emotional state;
- Walking by landing the toes first is more stable.

All of these points prove that it is crucial for our health to learn and to use the way of walking landing toes first.

7 | *Healthy Way of Walking Technique Details*

The healthy way of walking is based on good posture, and accordingly, its main points are the following:

- Good posture should be always maintained;
- Body weight should be kept on toes except while standing at ease. In addition, as T. Ellis noted "It is, however, hardly too much to say that, so long as the heel does reach the ground at every step, the less weight borne upon it, the better the walking." (T. Ellis, *The Human Foot*, p. 52);
- Toes should land first, beginning with the little toe (see details below);
- Position of rest should be naturally assumed by a foot just before the foot landing (see details below).

Note 1: Due to a number of unhealthy habits we have developed related to the way of walking by landing heels first, it is recommended to learn the healthy way of walking technique gradually. For instance, learn the proper standing technique first, because it includes the good posture technique described in the previous chapters. The standing technique is the basis for the next step, which is the ready-to-walk standing position, and consequently the later is the basis for the healthy way of walking. Then you can proceed with the walking on toes exercise and eventually with the complete healthy way of walking.

Note 2: You should be careful in the learning progress to make sure that the walking and standing techniques become more familiar, stable, and balanced in order to prevent any injuries (for instance, from loosing balance and falling, although that is very unlikely).

Note 3: If you feel tired while performing tests or techniques provided below, you should stop immediately and have a rest.

In a relaxed foot, the little toe is naturally in the lowest position and closest to the floor.

This notion is important for two reasons. First, it is a part of the natural healthy walking technique. Second, in this position a foot rests between steps. Let's look into details:

Test 1:

Raise your leg as shown in Fig. 22. For instance, do a short-to-medium sized step and then stop and relax the raised foot muscles. Note that at this point the toe is closer to the floor than the heel, and the little toe is in the lowest point. This is one more example showing that our bodies are naturally built with the ability to land toes first while walking and running.

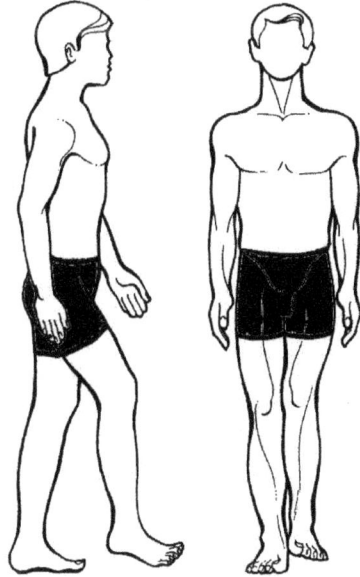

Fig. 22

In fact, you can note that *when you walk with short-to-medium steps landing heels first, you do some physical efforts (that pull your toes up) right before the foot landing.* Consequently your heels land first. In this connection, you can do one more interesting test.

Test 2:

Walk barefoot with short to medium steps and note the pulling toes up efforts.

In *The Human Foot* Thomas Ellis showed the Position of Rest, which also can be defined as position of relaxation as is depicted in Insert 6, Plate 8. He described the position of rest and its health benefits on p. 21 as follows:

Position of rest is the position to which the foot always tends in repose, and which it instinctively seeks when in pain. This I have elsewhere described, with reference to every part of the body, as one of the least stretching of the ligaments which bind the bones together, and most even adaptation of the joint surfaces to each other- of least tension and least pressure. This is always found in a mean between the extremes of motion. In respect of the ligaments collectively, one point of great importance should be noted. They share the influence of a law, universal in all the tissues of the body, that constant pressure or constant tension causes wasting, while intermittent pressure or intermittent tension promotes growth and strength, with, consequently, increased capacity for resistance. Thus if ligaments be constantly stretched as in prolonged and careless standing ... consequent deformity ensues. The words constant and intermittent are here used in their relative sense only. The rest which the night affords is not enough to counteract continuous strain during the day. When the stretching is absolutely constant, changes take place with great rapidity. On the other hand, when stretching and relaxation follow each other in frequent succession of changes and in great vigor, then the full effect in promoting growth is seen. Not only do the ligaments become stronger, but the attachments to the bones become more secure.

This explanation adds more health benefits to the way of walking landing toes first, because it includes the position of rest, which should be assumed by each foot for a fraction of a second right before the foot lands.

Base standing position

Assume good posture (see Figs. 14–16 for details). All body parts should be in balance. You should not fall forward or backward. All foot muscles are relaxed and out of tension, the body weight should be kept between toes and the middle of the feet, as opposed to placing most of the body weight on the heels as in the standing at ease position. In the beginning, you can stand at a wall (or a flat door) for a few minutes to get used to good posture (see Fig. 14). Later on you should be able to assume the posture without any wall.

Ready-to-walk standing position

In the beginning you might find this standing position uncomfortable. Later on, when you get used to it, you might reconsider the old habits of standing with poor posture as uncomfortable, and also you might feel then how unhealthy it was.

After you have assumed the base standing position described above, you can move to the ready-to-walk position as is shown in Fig. 23.

While still standing up in the base standing position, shift your body weight a little bit forward to your toes. Raise the chest completely up and let more air in. Pull in your stomach. Make sure you are still keeping the good posture and that all body parts are in balance. To check the balance, you can try to slowly rise to your toes. The body should not fall forward or backward.

Fig. 23

Walking on toes therapeutic exercise

The purpose of this exercise is to get used to walking by landing toes first assuming good posture. This is a must-know exercise before learning the complete healthy way of walking, because it includes around 90–95 percent of the walking landing toes first technique, but it is easier to perform. The exercise uses most of the healthy walking technique, it involves all of the necessary back muscle activity, and for that reason it should be considered as a *therapeutic walking exercise*. Also, it is the way of walking landing toes first tuning exercise. Even if you already use the healthy way of walking in your daily life or just as therapeutic walking, it is still recommended to perform the exercise on a regular basis. For instance, you could do it in the morning to warm up your muscles and tune up all related body parts to the healthy way of walking. Here is the exercise technique:

After assuming the ready-to-walk position (shown in Fig. 23), rise on your toes. Make sure that you still keep good posture. You might have to inhale a little bit more air and raise your chest slightly more up. This is the exercise base posture position and it should be kept for the whole work out.

Step forward with short-to-medium step length, landing the toe first beginning with the little toe. At the same time, keep the pushing leg straight and standing on its toe. Step with the other leg using the same technique. Continue walking, but do not land the heels at all during the whole exercise. In the beginning, it is recommended to walk on the toes for a minute or two. Every consequent time you can increase the time for one more minute. The more you do this exercise, the more you get used to the healthy way of walking technique. In addition, this exercise provides the same health benefits as the complete way of walking by landing toes first. Also, you will develop new healthy habits of walking that are necessary to go to the next step.

More details on the healthy way of walking technique:

The healthy way of walking technique combines all techniques described above, such us good posture, base standing position, ready-to-walk standing position, walking on toes exercise, and more. Let's look into more details.

1. Step length should be medium. The reason for medium length steps is that they are optimal. Short steps make the walking mincing. Long steps advance the legs too far, and consequently, the heels become the lowest to the ground point and land first. It breaks the whole technique and looses good posture. In Fig. 24 a short step sample is shown on the left, a long step is depicted in the middle, and the middle length step is located on the right.

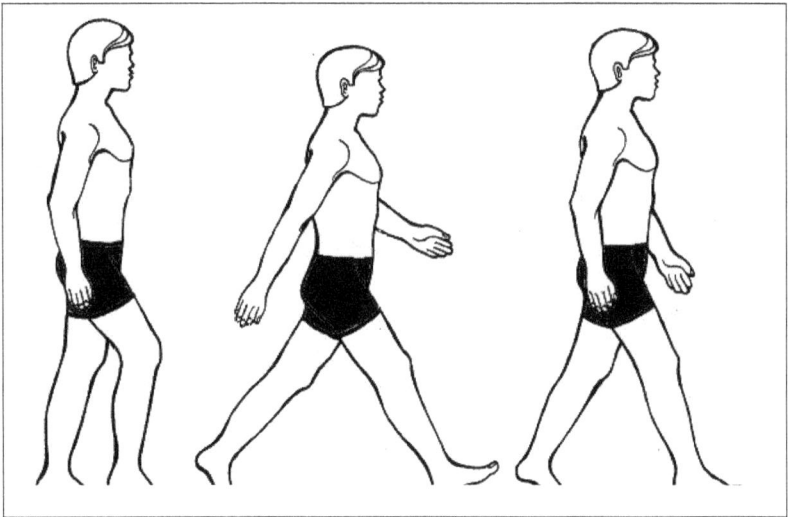

Fig. 24

2. Walking pace can be slow or moderate. It cannot be too fast. Unfortunately, in our contemporary lifestyle many people tend to walk fast, especially rushing to work. Tomas Ellis explained in *The Human Foot* on pp. 38 and 39: "In order that all movements, involved in a single step, should be done well, they must not be done

too rapidly. Fast walking, as done in foot-races, cannot possibly be done well; it ought not to be done at all. When an increase in speed is necessary, running is the natural course."

3. The pushing leg should be straight at the moment. After the push and before the landing, the advanced foot relaxes in the position of rest for a fraction of a second, and then when the foot is near the floor/ground, a slight tension appears as the shock absorbing effort. This technique works quite opposite to the way of walking by landing heels first, where no position of rest is assumed and some efforts are applied to the foot to pull the toes up (instead of relaxation) before the heel lands first.

4. The toe lands first beginning with the little toe, and momentarily the great toe, and then the heel lands. Similar technique has been described in *The Bodleys Afoot* book published in 1883. On p. 90 it is said: "When you change from foot to foot, the little toe should touch the ground first. Of course you won't walk on tip-toe, but the outer edge of the ball of the foot and the little toe will be on the ground first, and then the heel and the big toe; then when you push on, turn the foot, push from the inner edge of the ball of the foot, which should be the last to leave the ground. This sounds awkward, and if you were to try walking so, you would find yourself walking in a very clumsy manner; but, after practice, you would secure a steady and dignified gait." Another good reference can be found in the *British Manly Exercises* book published in 1834, on p. 9: "We have seen that, in the march, the toe externally first touches, and internally last leaves the ground."

5. Learning the healthy way of walking technique while barefooted is best. However, if you use shoes, shoes with no heels or shoes with low heels are preferable because high heels are more likely to land first.

6. The chest should be raised up to assume its full capacity (without any overdo), while the stomach should be pulled in. It helps to maintain good posture and provides other advantages described above. Having the chest at its full capacity, however, does not mean

that you should breathe excessively or fast. You should breathe just as much as you need.

7. Walk along an imaginable line that is optimal footprint patterns.

Note: This point is not critical, and it is provided here for the consistency only. In the first edition of this book, it was suggested that optimal footprint patterns (while walking along an imaginable line) are within a range between two patterns shown in Fig. 25 (see below).

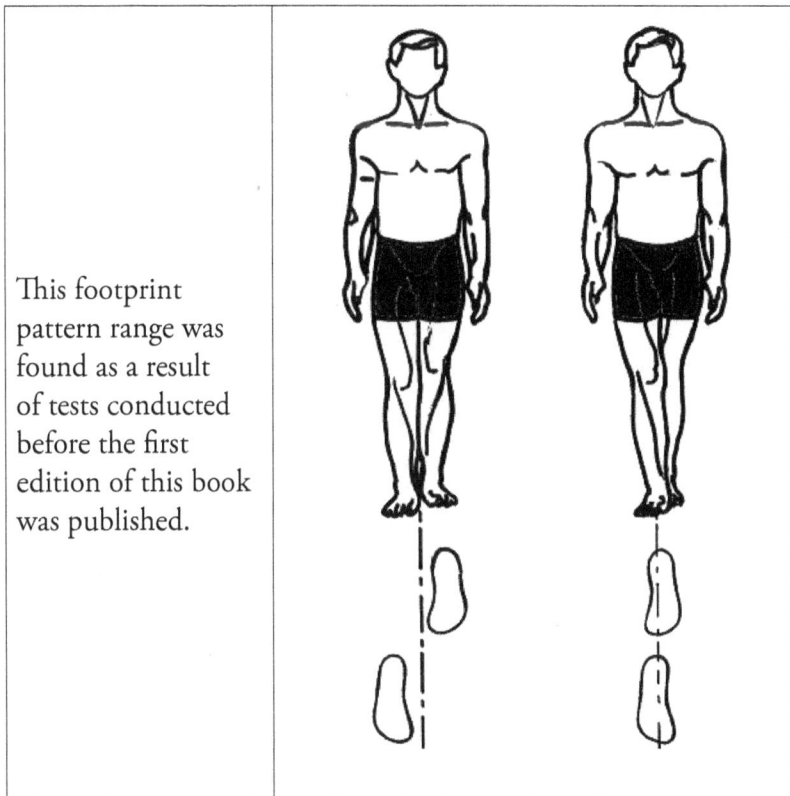

This footprint pattern range was found as a result of tests conducted before the first edition of this book was published.

Fig. 25

Later on when I came across the Thomas Ellis book, I found that his suggestion for the optimal footprint pattern is different, and this is the only point where his suggestion and mine did not come together. Why? Because there is no good scientific/medical reason for using any particular pattern and it seems to be a matter of personal preference. For instance, Thomas Ellis explained that a square is a firm shape and he recommended using it as a footprint pattern (*The Human Foot*, pp. 56–57).

However, for example, a triangle is known as a more firm shape, and actually it is believed to be the firmest. In addition, the shape approach might work for standing, but it does not make much sense for walking (as it explained below).

Here is what Thomas Ellis described about other opinions on the subject in the monograph on pp. 53–57:

I have before me a book on Calisthenics, where the author having prescribed an angle of 60 degrees, enjoins on the teacher to 'see that, while marching, the pupils point their toes down.' As to turning out the toes, Camper was very emphatic. He said that it was 'incontestable,' for the reason 'that we then form with the two feet a kind of triangle, which, like the tripod, gives them firmness.' The poet, on the contrary, tells us of 'A tower that stood four square to every wind that blew.' And the expression standing square to all four winds of heaven is familiar, as indicative of the firmness of a structure.

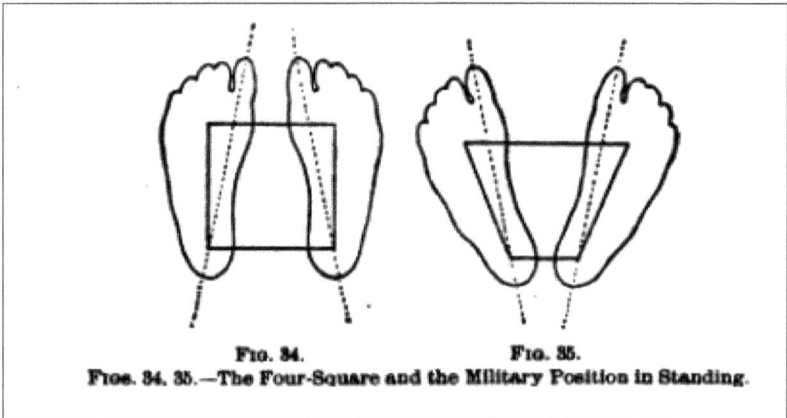

Fig. 34.   Fig. 35.
Figs. 34, 35.—The Four-Square and the Military Position in Standing.

T. Ellis, Figs. 34, 35

Thomas Ellis provided more details: "The four square position should be maintained for walking. In Fig. 36 [see below] each foot is in precisely the same relation to the line along which the body is supposed to be moving as, in Fig. 34, it is to one between the two. The importance of Meyer's line, here indicated dots, has already been mentioned." (*The Human Foot*, p. 68)

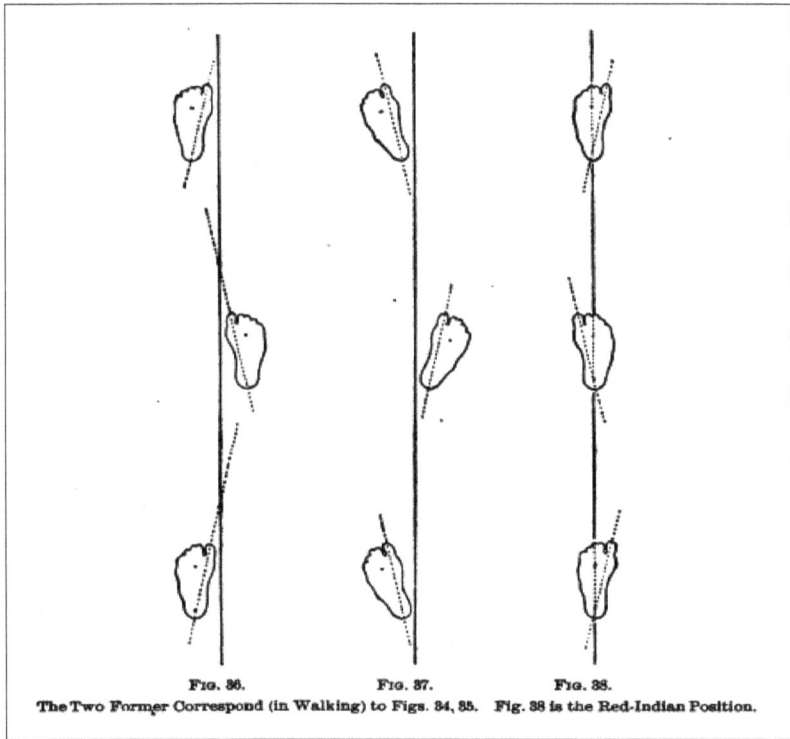

FIG. 36.   FIG. 37.   FIG. 38.
The Two Former Correspond (in Walking) to Figs. 34, 35.   Fig. 38 is the Red-Indian Position.

T. Ellis, Figs. 36–38

To understand this approach better, we need to look into the four-square position and the Meyer's line description Thomas Ellis provided in *The Human Foot* on p. 9:

Professor Meyer, of Zurich, more than thirty years ago pointed out the important fact that, in a natural, healthy foot the middle line of the great toe continued backward passes through a central point in the heel. He might, I think, have gone further, and said that all the toes radiate from that centre. This line, which should always be called Meyer's line, is shown in Pl. 7, Fig. 20. This plate is taken from a foot-print made by a foot, the sole of which had been covered with printer's ink, and drawn in duplicate.

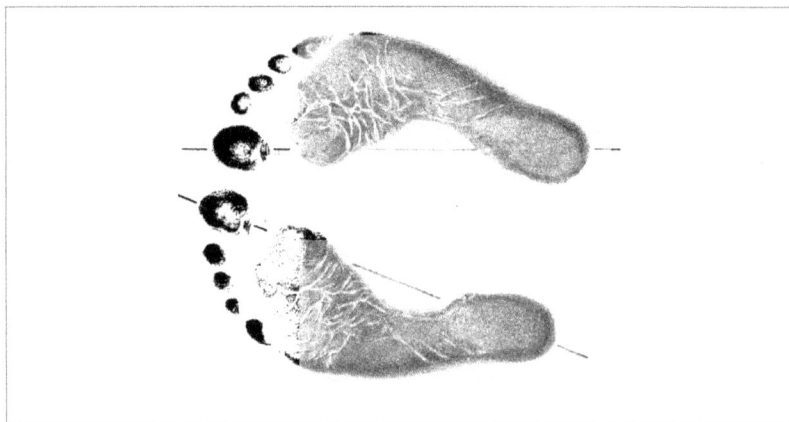

T. Ellis, Plate 7, Fig 20

Meyer's line being on the sole is not, under ordinary conditions, visible, but more than this, it has no surface mark to indicate its position. If, however, we continue the middle of the great toe on the upper surface backward to the ankle, we find that it runs along the highest part of the foot; it runs, in fact, along the crest of the ridge. Here we have something tangible, visible. This is a line to which reference may be made in studying the contour of the foot.] (T. Ellis, p. 9

Please note, that Military Position and the Camper's position are two more approaches, and they are different from two others mentioned before. Following is the military position in walking description found in *British Manly Exercises*, p. 8:

The head should be upright, easy, and capable of free motion, right, left, up, or down, without affecting the position of the body. The latter should be upright, having the breast projected, and the stomach retracted, though not so as to injure either freedom or respiration, or ease of attitude. The shoulders should be kept moderately and equally back and low; and the arms should hang unconstrainedly by the sides. The knees should be straight; the toes should form nearly half a right angle with the line of the walk; and the weight of the body should rest principally on the balls of the feet.

I tested the Thomas Ellis suggested footprint patterns well as other recommendations and found that the patterns, which could be placed somewhere between those shown on T. Ellis, Fig. 36 and Fig. 37 (see below) also work fine for me. That is why I believe that all optimal footprint pattern recommendations should not be taken as rules. They are only suggestions, and the best footprint pattern with the most convenient foot angle to the imaginable line should be found on an individual basis.

8. Slippers, flip-flops and similar shoes should be avoided whenever possible; at least the use of them should be minimized, as they require pulling your toes up while walking to keep them on. Otherwise, they just fall off the feet if the toes point downward. The pulling toes up efforts break the whole healthy walking technique, because you would have to land your feet on your heels first with all unhealthy consequences, such as automatically assuming poor posture.

When it comes to using something new and unusual, for instance, walking by landing toes first, most people might hesitate, thinking about their appearance while learning the new techniques, even though they know this way of walking is healthier. That is why the aesthetics should be considered.

In the "good old times" the way of walking by landing toes first was associated with graciousness. Let's look into some interesting quotes from Alexandre Dumas's *The Three Musketeers*. In chapter XII *George Villiers, Duke of Buckingham* the author describes: "Anna of Austria was then from twenty-six or twenty-seven years of age, that is to say, she was in the full splendor of her beauty. Her carriage was that of a queen or a goddess ...." [Dumas, A., *The Three Musketeers* (Translated by Robson W.), p. 83.]

In the same book in chapter VII *The Interior of "The Musketeers,"* the author compares two musketeers Athos and Porthos: "with his simple musketeer's uniform and nothing but the manner in which he threw back his head and advanced his foot, Athos instantly took the place which was his due, and consigned the ostentatious Porthos to the second rank." [Dumas, A., *The Three Musketeers* (Translated by Robson W.), p. 49.]

Famous ancient Greek philosopher Pythagoras hardly admitted new students to his classes, pointing out that "not every piece of wood is good for curving out Mercury." In a candidate evaluation procedure he paid close attention to the youths' laughter and way of walking, as it was described in the *Les Grands Inities* book by Edouard Schure.

Sophia Voskresenskaya explained the aesthetics of posture and different ways of walking in her book *The Hostess Friend published in 1909*:

Regardless of how beautiful is a personal appearance, nobody can leave a good impression if the person's posture and way of walking do not correspond with each other and don't match the person's figure. Such violation of harmony also damages our dignity.

Posture and way of walking are very important subjects. However, they should be taken in moderation. Good posture should not be unmovable and stiff. On the other hand, a posture that is too relaxed and loose, or that requires you to lean on your elbows is not well-mannered …

A person's walk always displays his or her character. Some people are recognized by their way of walking even before their faces are recognized. For this reason, our ways of walking deserve close attention. Harmony is also a motto for walking. You should never step landing the whole foot, let alone landing the heel first. The first is rude, and the second is a bad manner. You should always step landing toes first; only then the foot will acquire a steep curve and look elegant, and the way of walking will become graceful. However, you should not go to extremes like hopping or sort of dancing while walking because it looks ridiculously affected. A gliding walk enchanted by poets in the past and glorified by novelists, was considered to be an attribute of charming femininity, but is it possible to do it in the modern world? Unfortunately, a gliding walk is out of fashion. Contemporary style requires firm steps which characterizes the current independent status of females. However, it would be much better if this independence wouldn't apply to their walk and would have a better use than loud footsteps.

Thomas Ellis in *The Human Foot* on p. 91 provided an interesting point of view about high heels and the aesthetics pertaining to ways of walking.

High heels are supposed to be an elegance derived from the French … It is not, however, generally recognized that the French idea of a high heel is a thing to rest on, not to walk on. The observant Max O'Rell, who has contrasted the manners and customs of the two countries, says that an English lady walks with her arms hanging down, supporting herself on her heels; the French lady walks with her arms bent, supporting herself on the toes. I have seen it stated, in print and in all gravity, that French ladies actually practice this manner of walking with a slipper fitted with an India-rubber ball beneath the heel. This ball squeaks when subjected to pressure, and the object in the practice is to move freely and yet not sound this squeak.

Another interesting aesthetic point Tomas Ellis brought up is that the way of walking by landing toes first forms the shape of legs better. On p. 38 he explained:

Under the influence of vigorous and rapidly executed movements, the muscles of the calf and lower part of the leg are modified in form, as well as increased in size. The fleshy (muscular) fibers of the deeper muscles [see Insert 7, Plate 3, Fig. 8] are extended very much lower than those of the calf muscles, where the tendon extends high up into the leg. Thus an enlargement takes place just above the ankle, gently increasing to the calf... Thus development depends not only on the amount but on the manner of the exercise. Excellence of form depends on exercise of junction and on the manner in which function is fulfilled. This is true of the foot as regards strength as well as beauty, and if it be admitted then will be recognized the importance of properly performing the most ordinary functions. Foremost among these are standing and walking; but as we are discussing movements the latter will be taken first.

Thomas Ellis expressed how he was astounded with the human foot structure. In *The Human Foot* on p. 17 he noted that "more human foot is studied, more absolute perfection of its mechanism is evident." In fact, in this book further research was presented on the subject of the next step. That is, that the way of walking by landing toes first (which is physically possible because of the foot built-in digitigrade mechanism) does provide the ability to maintain good posture, which can be called perfection as well, because it combines the best aesthetic appearance and health benefits.

9 | *Exercises*

It is recommended that exercises provided in this chapter be performed on a regular basis—preferably in the morning to work out and strengthen back and other muscles. Also, exercises 1 and 2 tune the body for using good posture and the healthy way of walking in daily life.

Please note: For certain medical conditions, for instance, a cracked spinal disk, it might not be recommended to perform some exercises. In such cases, consult your doctor. Also, if any uncomfortable feeling occurs while performing the exercises, you should stop and let your muscles rest. A steady learning pace is recommended.

Your doctor might provide you with more exercises. In addition, you can find many of them at the American Chiropractic Association website at http://www.amerchiro.org.

In my case, I used the set of exercises provided below (together with the healthy way of walking) to cure my lower, mid, and upper chronic back pain.

The exercises shown below can be performed by both men and women. You should start with a couple of exercises (for instance, the first and second), and then add one more exercise at a time. It is recommended to repeat exercises for three to four times in the beginning, and then you can do more repetitions later on. Also, you should do exercises slowly at first, and then you can gradually speed them up. To avoid any injury, you should not overstretch yourself while doing the exercises. On the contrary, try to do them with ease, and stop immediately if you feel any awkwardness or pain.

1. Stand at the wall, assuming good posture for one to three minutes as shown in Fig. 26. The standing at the wall exercise technique has been described in detail in Chapter 5.

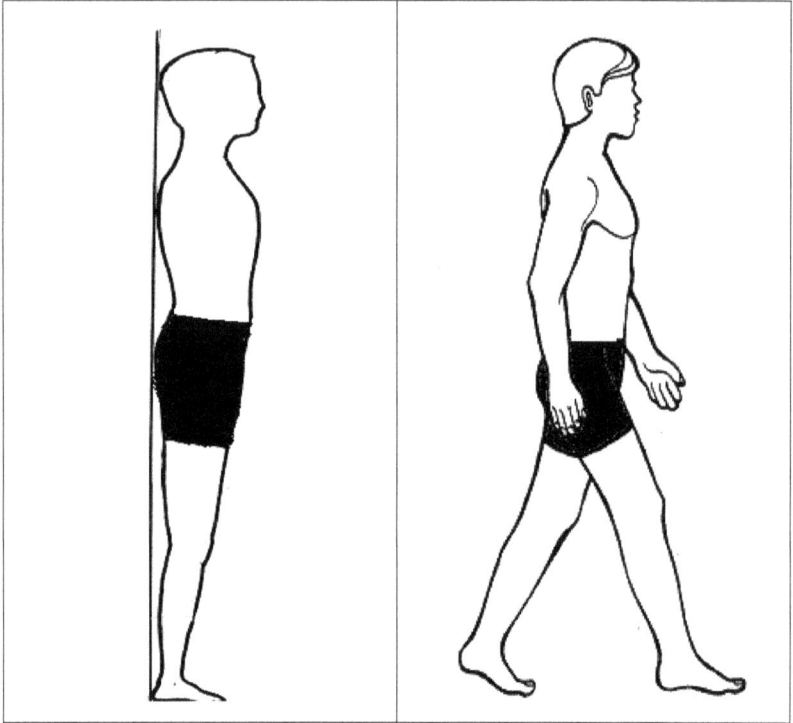

Fig.26   Fig.27

2. Walk on the toes (no stepping on heels at all) using the healthy way of walking landing toes first technique for one to ten minutes, as shown in Fig. 27. The walking on toes exercise could be performed barefooted or in shoes. Most important is to keep good posture while walking. This exercise provides all health benefits related to the healthy way of walking as described in previous chapters. In other words, it has curing qualities, and that is why it sometimes referred to as *therapeutic walking exercise*. This exercise is one of the best for learning and keeping up the healthy way of walking technique, and therefore it should be performed on a regular basis.

In addition, it is recommended to use it in daily life whenever possible to get most of the related health benefits. The exercise detailed description can be found in Chapter 7.

3. The exercise shown in Fig. 28 helps to train the vertebrae flexibility, and also works out and strengthens back muscles. Please note: At step 2 from the lowest point, you should rise several inches up and sit down one more time.

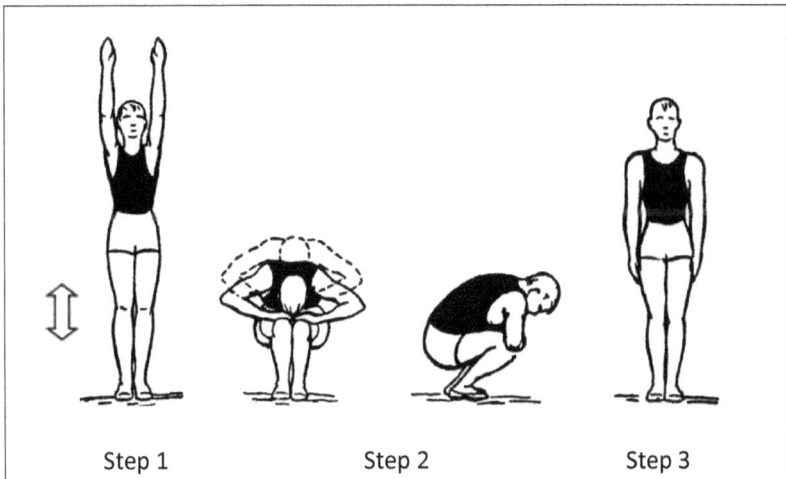

Fig. 28

4. The exercise shown in Fig. 29 works out and strengthens back muscles more to be able to maintain good posture and secure the vertebrae. For this reason, the exercise should be performed anywhere from –three to four times in the beginning, and up to one hundred times later on.. This is one of the best back muscle training exercises. For instance, when I was dealing with back pain, my doctor advised me of the value of repeating this exercise up to one hundred times. However, you should not overstretch yourself while performing the exercise. On the contrary, you should do it with ease gradually increasing the number of repetitions. Touching the floor is optional. Another option is to hold hands behind head and keep elbows apart while performing the exercise (same way as is shown in Fig. 35).

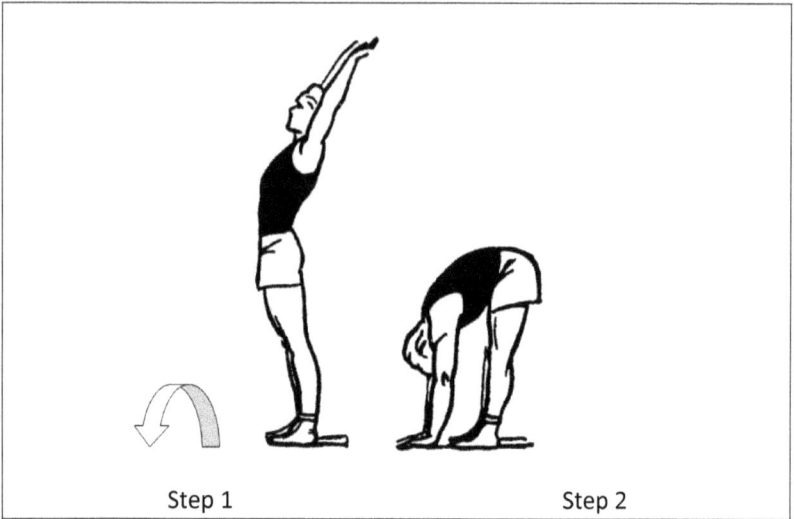

Step 1   Step 2

Fig. 29

5. The exercise shown in Fig. 30 is also one of the best back muscle exercises, because it trains the muscles that act upon vertebrae twisting movements. The condition of these muscles is critical for securing the vertebrae.

Lie down on the floor and extend your arms to both sides, palms face down. Stretch your legs and raise them up to make a right angle between your body and your legs as shown in Fig. 30, Step 1. Slowly move your legs down to the left until they touch the floor, keeping the right angle as shown in Step 2. Then, slowly raise the legs back up as shown in step 3, still keeping the right angle. After that, slowly move your legs down to the right until they touch the floor still keeping the angle right as shown in step 4. Return legs to Step 1 position.

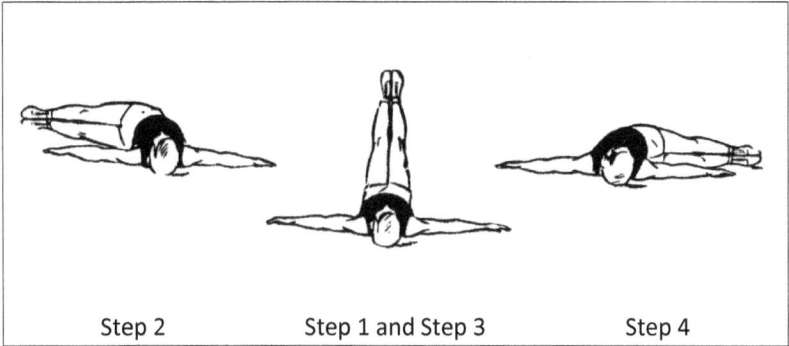

Step 2   Step 1 and Step 3   Step 4

Fig. 30

6. The exercises shown in Figs. 31–33 work out back muscles and train vertebrae flexibility. Start with the exercise shown in Fig. 31.

Bend to the left twice. Then bend to the right couple times. Do not lean your head or the body forward or backward.

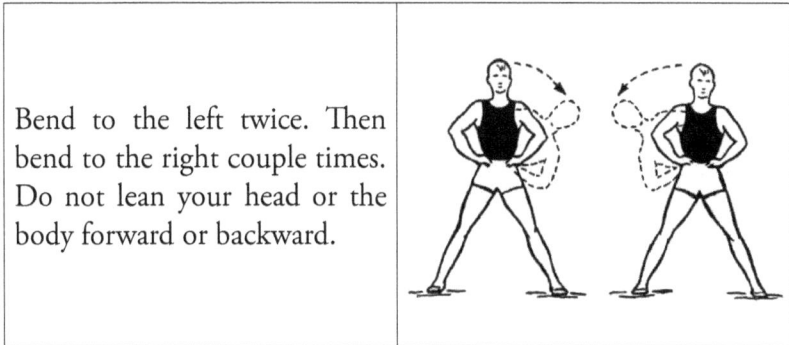

Fig. 31

Modify the exercise as is shown in Fig. 32 by bending one knee at a time, which extends the flexing.

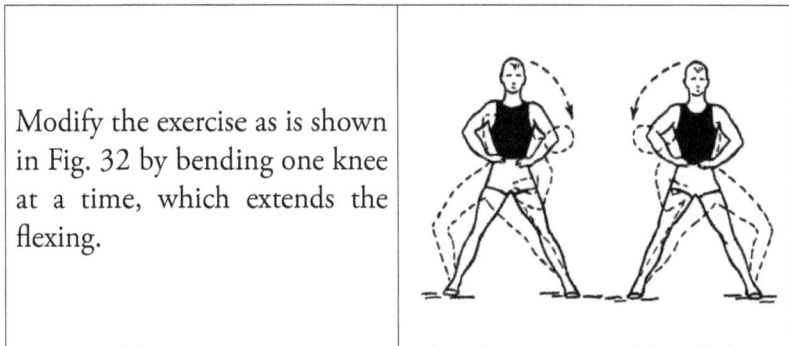

Fig. 32

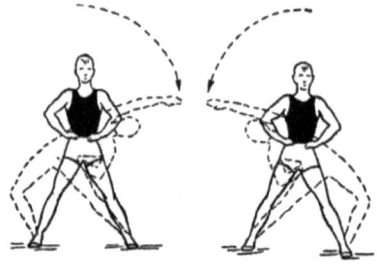

The exercise shown in Fig. 33 extends flexing further by adding a raised arm to the bending knee at the same time.

Fig. 33

7. The exercise shown in Fig. 34 combines twisting, bending, and rotating torso movements. Steps 1–5 in Fig. 34 illustrate how to perform it with the right arm. It should be done the same way for the left arm.

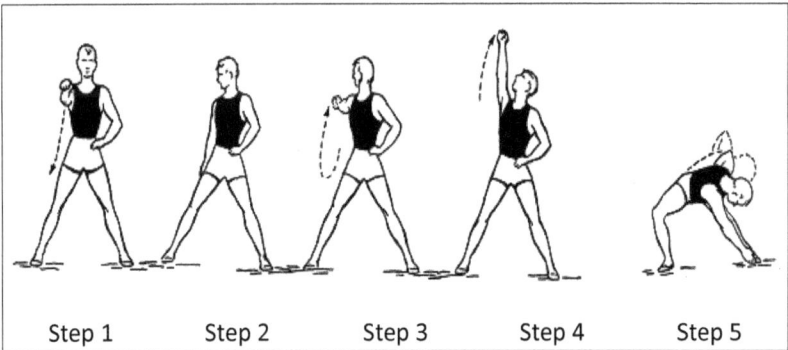

| Step 1 | Step 2 | Step 3 | Step 4 | Step 5 |

Fig. 34

Exercises 8 and 9 are shown in Fig. 35 and Fig. 36 respectively. They are based on body rotating movements. The exercises work out back muscles and train the vertebrae to become more flexible.

8a. Stand straight up, keeping your feet together. Put your arms on the back of your head (you can interlock fingers), extending elbows to the sides. First, rotate your pelvis in one direction four to eight times, holding your shoulders in the same place as is shown in Fig. 35 Steps 1 and 2. Then do it in the opposite direction.

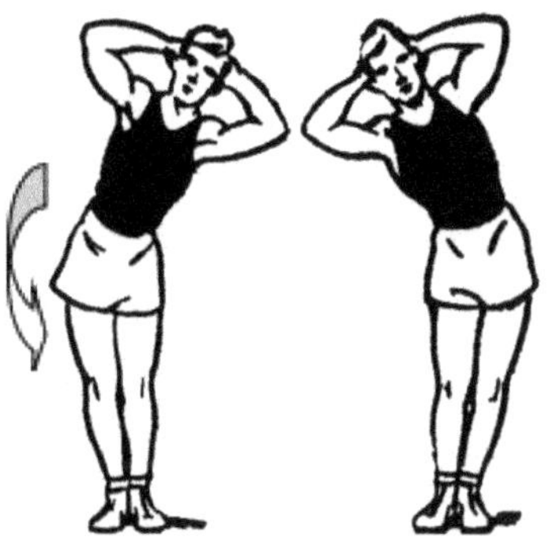

Step 1   Step 2

Fig. 35

8b. Stand, keeping feet one short step aside as wide as your shoulders. Do the same rotations in both directions.

9. The exercise shown in Fig. 36 is similar to the previous one. The difference is that you should hold your pelvis in place and rotate your torso only. First, do it in one direction and then in the opposite.

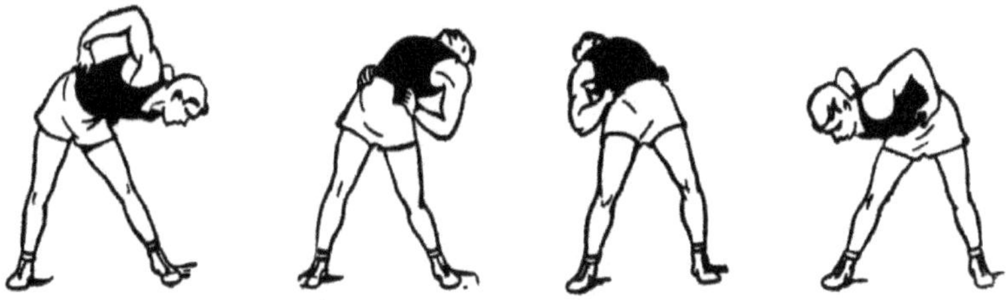

Step 1   Step 2   Step 3   Step 4

Fig. 36

Exercises 10 and 11 are shown in Figs. 37 and 38 respectively. They designed to work out and train hip joints and muscles, which are critical for proper walking.

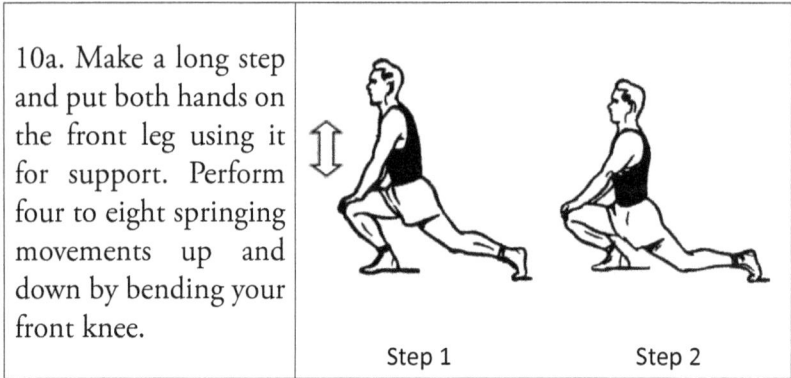

10a. Make a long step and put both hands on the front leg using it for support. Perform four to eight springing movements up and down by bending your front knee.

Step 1   Step 2

Fig. 37

10b. Make a long step with the other leg (or turn over) and perform four to eight springing movements for the other leg.

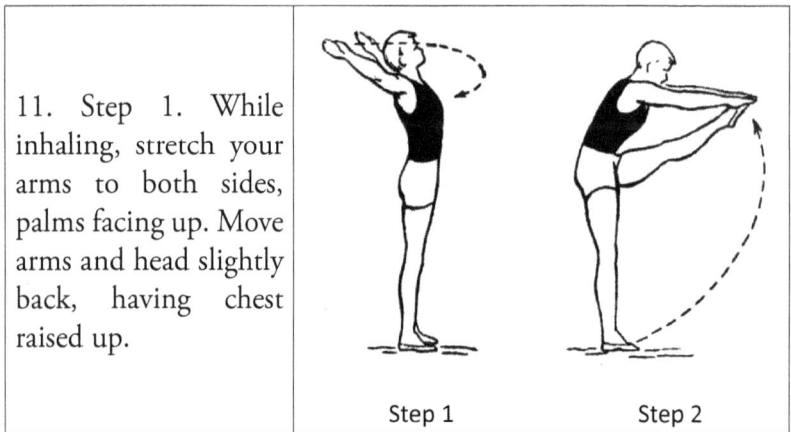

11. Step 1. While inhaling, stretch your arms to both sides, palms facing up. Move arms and head slightly back, having chest raised up.

Step 1   Step 2

Fig. 38

Step 2. While exhaling, move straight arms to the front, turning palms down. Simultaneously raise one leg up, keeping it straight.

Slightly nod the head down towards to the raised leg. Then return the head, arms, and the leg back to Step 1. After that, perform Step 2 using the other leg. It is not recommended to raise legs too high. You should not overstretch yourself.

12. The exercise shown in Fig. 39 is designed to help you catch your breath after performing the exercises described above. Stand up, keeping your feet apart as shown in Step 1. At Step 2 while inhaling slowly rise to your toes. Simultaneously raise your arms, palms facing up. At Step 3, while exhaling, descend to your feet, cross your relaxed arms in front of you, and bend down slightly. Repeat the exercise three to four times.

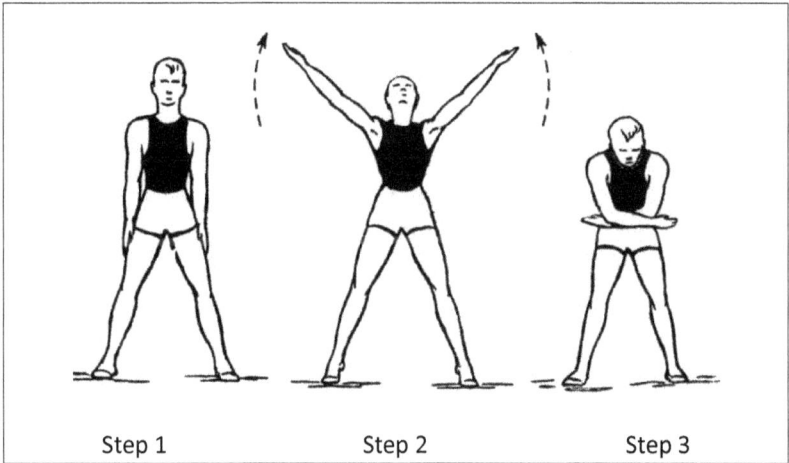

Step 1   Step 2   Step 3

Fig. 39

INSERT 1

Vertebrae misalignment

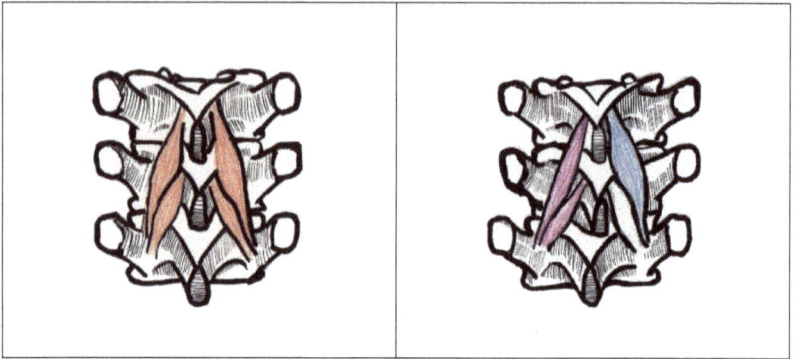

Fig. 2   Fig. 3

The misalignment strains and stretches left side muscles (shown in purple in Fig. 3). On the right side it causes muscles (shown in blue) to shrink to the shorter distance, and possibly to wrench. This type of muscle stretching and wrenching causes back pain.

Vertebrae disk dehydration.

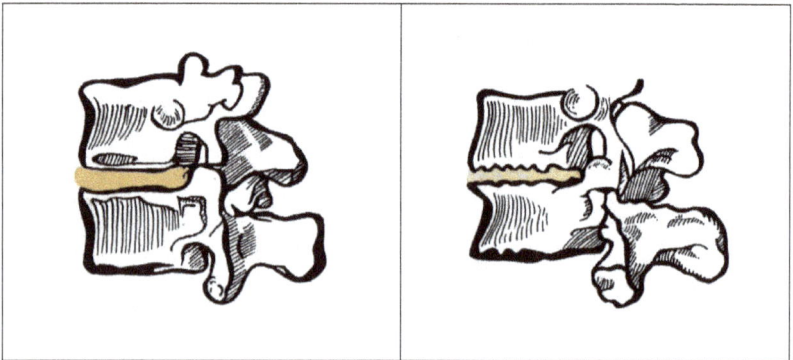

Fig. 6   Fig. 7

One of many possible back pain causes is spinal disk dehydration. Each spinal disk contains some fluid. Fig. 6 shows a normally hydrated spinal disk. When there is not enough fluid in the disk to keep it hydrated, it causes back pain, as is shown in Fig. 7.

INSERT 2

Pinched or irritated nerve roots can cause pain and other problems in related organs depending on what particular nerve root is involved.

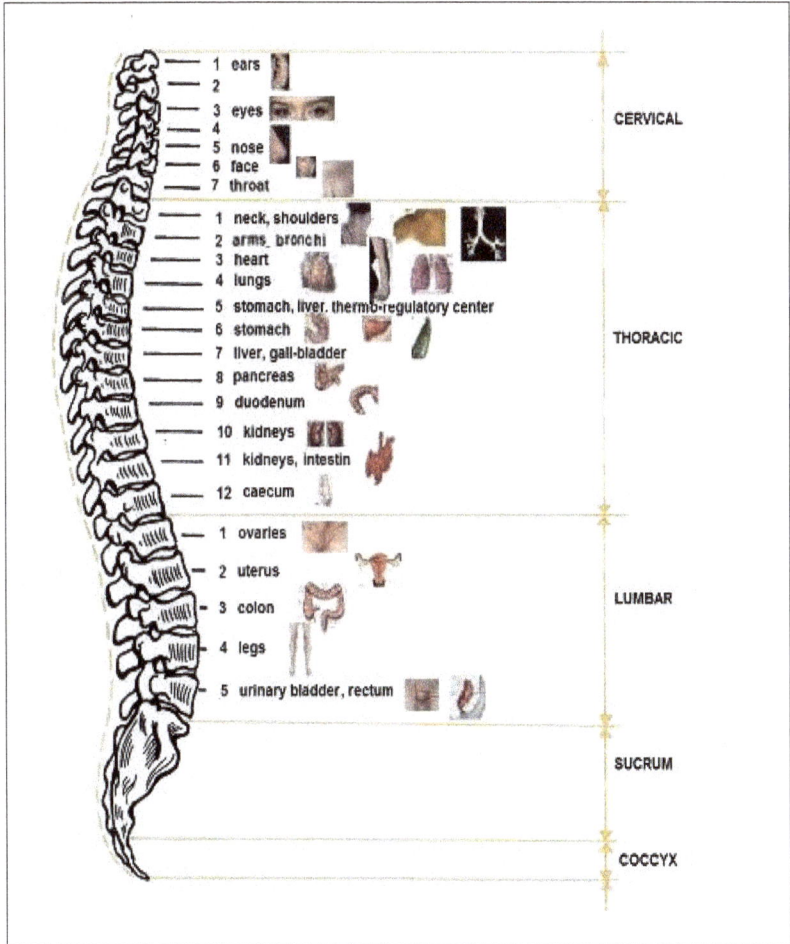

Fig. 4

INSERT 3

Back muscles support vertebrae from all sides

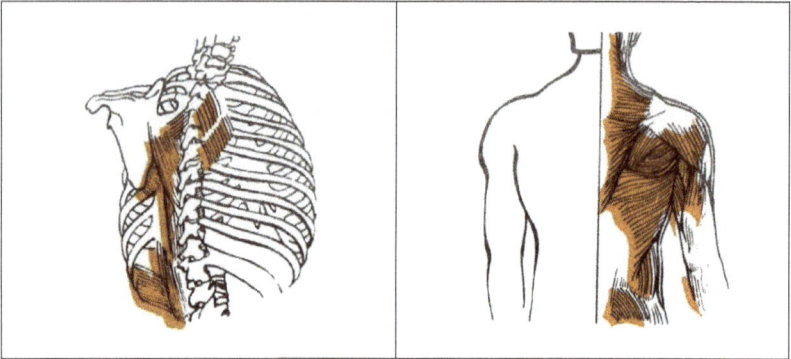

Fig. 8   Fig. 9

In Fig.8 and Fig.9 it is shown that back muscles naturally cover the vertebrae. When the muscles are strong, they are able to secure the back bones and spinal disks in their proper locations.

Muscle activities assist blood circulation

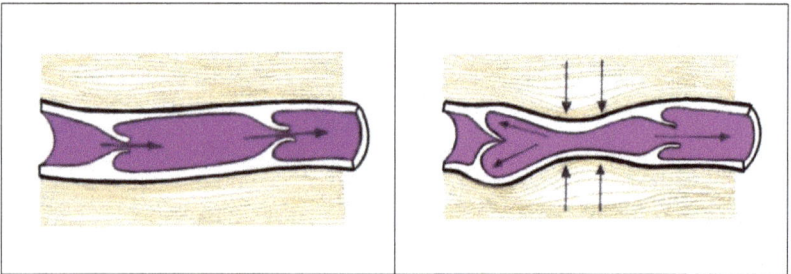

Fig. 10   Fig. 11

First, the heart pumps out a portion of blood into arteries toward all organs and muscles. However, these efforts are enough just to bring fresh nutrients and oxygen to body cells. The cells return back into the blood their waist products and carbon dioxide. After that process blood goes into veins, for example, as it is depicted for one vain in Fig. 10. When the surrounding muscles flex, they squeeze the vein as is shown in Fig. 11. That pushes blood to both directions, but the blood vessels have inner valves that allow the flow to go one way only back to the heart.

INSERT 4

Lumbar curve

Who benefits from poor posture? This is only the stomach, because it freely expands forward. However, it also pulls the lower vertebrae (lumbar shown in Fig. 17) out of its normal position (shown in Fig. 18), giving it a sharper curve as is shown in Fig. 19. This sharp curve makes the lumbar more vulnerable to vertebrae misalignments and spinal disk slips.

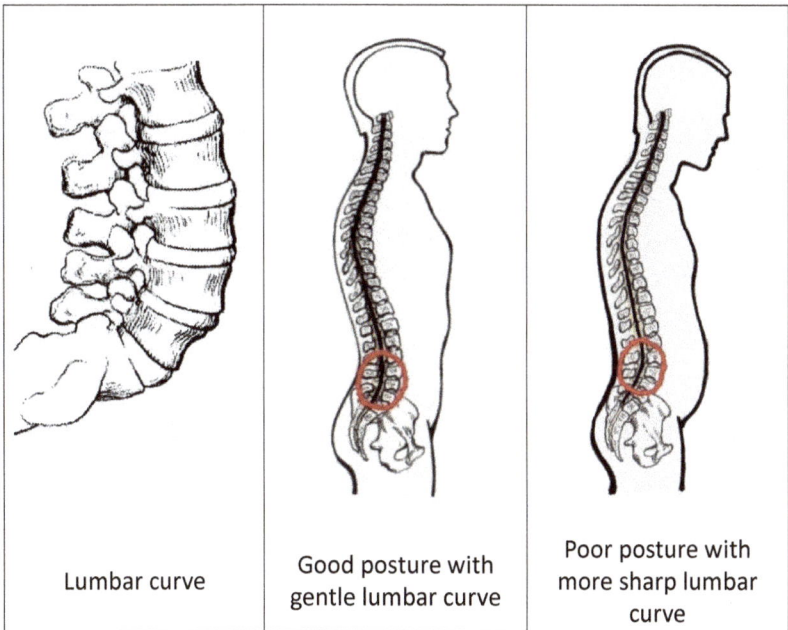

Lumbar curve	Good posture with gentle lumbar curve	Poor posture with more sharp lumbar curve
Fig. 17	Fig. 18	Fig. 19

INSERT 5

Rising to toes mechanism built-in to human foot

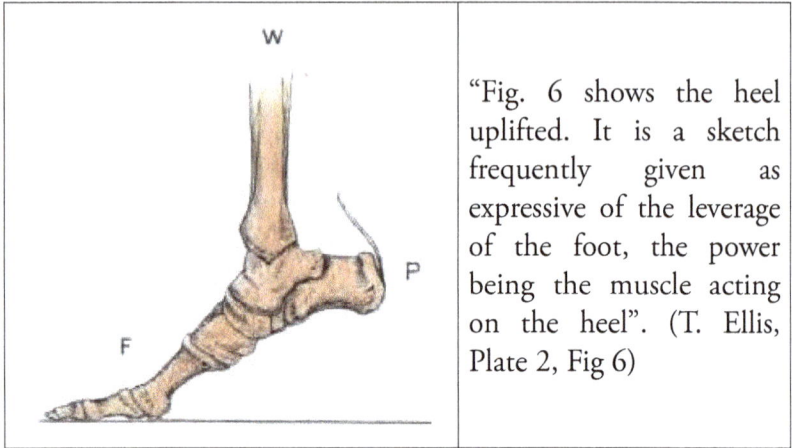

"Fig. 6 shows the heel uplifted. It is a sketch frequently given as expressive of the leverage of the foot, the power being the muscle acting on the heel". (T. Ellis, Plate 2, Fig 6)

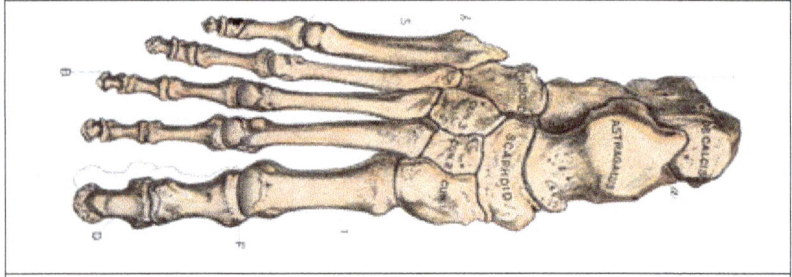

"Fig. 1 is a view of the upper surface of the skeleton of the right foot". (T. Ellis, Plate 1, Fig. 1)

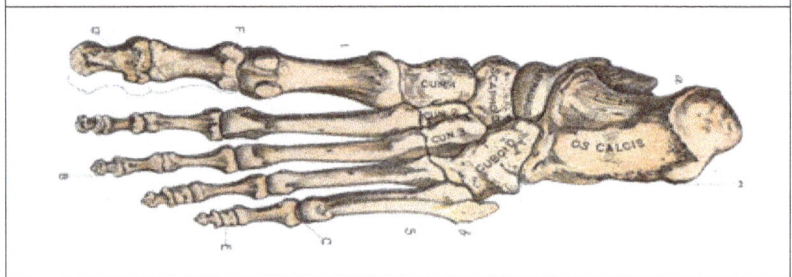

"Fig 2 shows the same (right) foot turned over and the under surface seen." (T. Ellis, Plate 2, Fig. 2)

INSERT 6

Foot arch

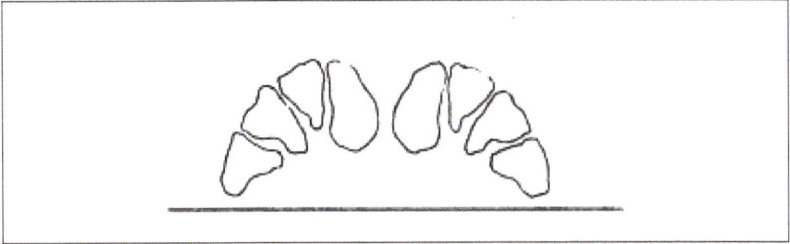

"Fig. 3 is a section, in outline, of the three cuneiform and of the cuboid bones, taken obliquely across each foot. It marks a transverse *arch* in each foot, the two combining to form a larger arch." (T. Ellis, Plate 1, Fig. 3)

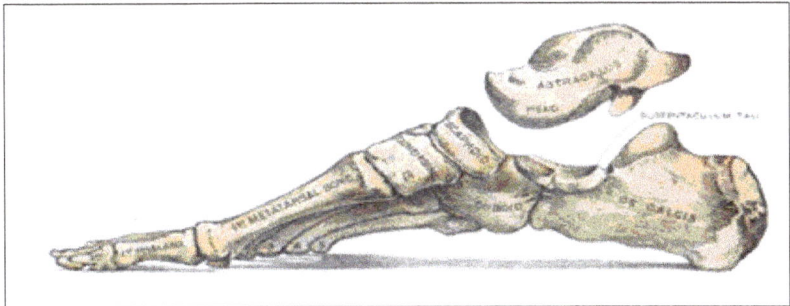

"Fig. 11 is a view of the bones forming the *arch* of the foot seen from the inner side." (T. Ellis, Plate 4, Fig. 11)

Position of rest

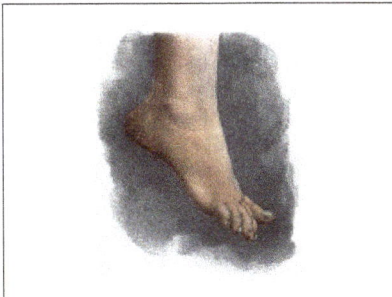

"Position of rest."
(T. Ellis, Plate 8)

INSERT 7

Foot strong ligaments

"Fig. 5 shows how the bones of the tarsus, seen on the inner margin, are bound to the leg bone, to the metatarsus and to each other by strong ligaments." (T. Ellis, Plate 2, Fig. 5)

"Fig. 8 gives a view, so far as can be seen from the inner side." (T. Ellis, Plate 3, Fig. 8)

"Fig. 15 is the outer view corresponding to Fig. 8." (T. Ellis, Plate 5, Fig. 15)

"Fig. 9 is a view as given by a division of the foot through the joints immediately in front of the ankle." (T. Ellis, Plate 3, Fig. 9)

"Fig. 16 is a vertical, transverse section through the ankle." (T. Ellis, Plate 5, Fig. 16)

INSERT 8

Three layers of muscles as seen in the upturned sole

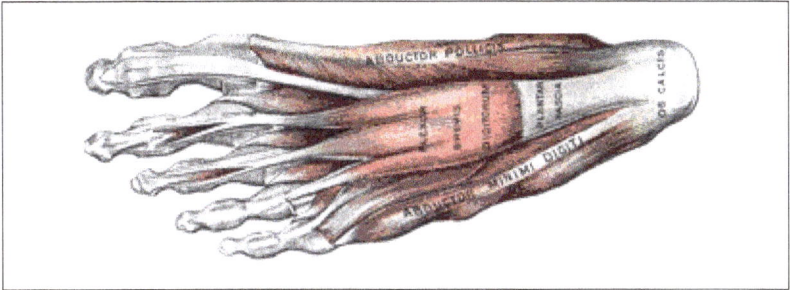

"Fig 7 represents the first or the most superficial layer of the muscles seen in the upturned sole." (T. Ellis, Plate 3, Fig. 7)

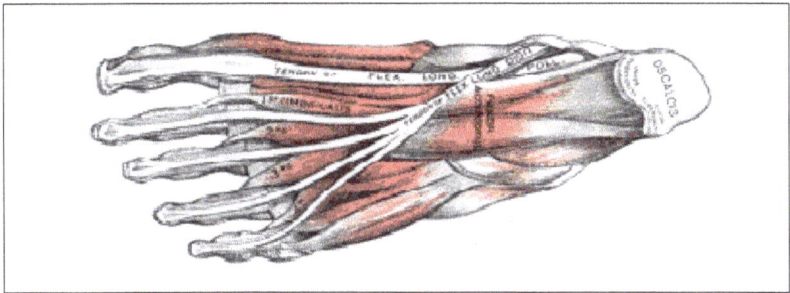

"Fig 7 represents the first or the most superficial layer of the muscles seen in the upturned sole." (T. Ellis, Plate 3, Fig. 7)

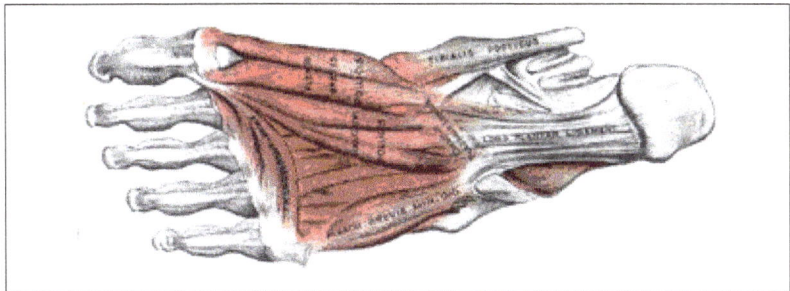

"Fig 7 represents the first or the most superficial layer of the muscles seen in the upturned sole." (T. Ellis, Plate 3, Fig. 7)

BIBLIOGRAPHY

Alexseev A. *Science and Life.* Moscow, 24 Miasnitzkaya St., 1979, #4 [Алексеев А. Наука и Жизнь. Москва, Мясницкая ул. , д. 24, 1973, No. 4]

Danford, Howard Gorby. *Creative Leadership in Recreation.* Published by Allyn and Bacon, 1964

Dumas, Alexandre. *The Three Musketeers.* (Translated by William Robson), George Routledge and Co., Farringdon St., London, 1853.

Ellis, Thomas S. M.R.C.S. *The Human Foot: Its Form and Structure, Functions and Clothing.* Wood's Medical and Surgical Monographs. William Wood and Company Publishers, New York, Volume 6 Number 1, April 1890.

Gore, R. *The First Steps.* National Geographic, Feb. 1997.

Halfpenny, James C., Biesiot. A. Elizabeth. *Field Guide to Mammal Tracking in North America.* Johnson Books, 1986.

Herbert, W. *Was Lucy a Climber? Dissenting Views of Ancient Bones. Science News, Vol. 122, No. 8, Aug. 21, 1982.*

Hopple, Christine J. *Teaching for Outcomes in Elementary Physical Education.* Published by Human Kinetics, 1995.

Johanson, Donald C. and Blake Edgar. *Face-to-Face with Lucy's Family.* National Geographic #189, 1996.

Johanson, Donald et al. *Lucy the Beginning of Humankind.* Science, 1981.

Kalverboer, Alex F. at all. *Handbook of Brain and Behavior in Human Development.* Kluwer Academic Publishers, 1993.

Leakey Mary D. et al. *Pleocene Footprints in the Laetolil Beds at Laetoli, Northern Tanzania.* Nature Vol. 278, Mar. 22, 1978.

Meyers, Casey. *Walking: A Complete Guide to the Complete Exercise.* Published by Random House, 1992.

Nagel, Charles, Moore Fredricka. *Skill Development Through Games and Rhythmic Activities.* National Press, 1966.

Nordemar, R. *Back Pain* (translated from Sweden). Moscow: Medicine, 1991. (Нордемар Р. Боль в Спине: Пер. с швед. М.:Медицина, 1991.)

Pica, Rae. *Your Active Child*, The McGraw-Hill Companies, 2003.

Research Intelligence. University of Liverpool. # 22, Nov. 2004

Romanes, George John, M.A., LL.D, F.R.S. *Darwin and After Darwin.* Chicago, The Open Court Publishing Company, 1910.

Scudder, Horace Elisha. *The Bodleys Afoot.* Boston Houghton, Mifflin and Co., 1883.

Searfoss Glen. Skulls and Bones: *A Guide to the Skeletal Structures and Behavior of North American Mammals.* Stackpole Books, 1995.

Schure, Eduard. *Great Initiates.* (Fr. Schure Edouard. Les Grands Inities.) (Translated from French), Published by TGZU Kaluga 1914. [Шюре Э. Великие Посвясчённые: Пер. с фр. Калуга: Тип. Губерн. Зем. Управы, 1914].

The Lucy Link. Time. Jan. 29, 1979.

Vesalius, Andreaes. *De Humani Corporis Fabrica.* Basel: J. Oporinus, 1543.

Voskresenskaya, Sophia. *The Hostess Friend.* A.A. Kaspary Publications, 1909. [Воскресенская С. И. Друг Хозяйки. СПб: Изд-во А.А. Каспари, 1909.]

Walker, Donald. *British Manly Exercises: Containing Rowing and Sailing, Riding & Driiving.* Philadelphia: Thomas Wardle, 15 Minor Street, 1836.

Walker, Donald. *British Manly Exercises.* T. Hurst, 65 Pauls Church Yard, London, 1834.

Wong, Kate. *Footprints to Fill.* Scientific American, August 1, 2005.

Yanker, Gary. *Walkshaping: Indoors or Out, 6 Weeks to a Better Body.* Hearst Books, 1995.

Art images used on the front cover from left to right and from top to bottom:

Tobias and the Angel, painting by Andrea del Verrocchio;
Primavera, painting by Sandro Botticelli;
Hermes (The Flying Mercury), statue by Giovanni Da Bologna;
A prehistoric Saharan rock art;
Pompeii Art, Fresco from the Villa of the Mysteries; Atalanta, statue by Pierre Lepautre.

Art images used on the back cover from left to right and from top to bottom:

Achilles and Penthesilea (an ancient Greek painting on a big platter);
The Birth of Venus, painting by Sandro Botticelli; David, statue by Michelangelo;
The Feast of Venus, painting by Peter Paul Rubens.

www.ingramcontent.com/pod-product-compliance
Lightning Source LLC
Chambersburg PA
CBHW052119030426
42335CB00025B/3051